The Mindset of Weight Loss

"Transform Your Mindset, Transform Your Body: The Key to Lasting Weight Loss Success"

PUBLISHED BY:

Anthony Ezigbo

Copyright Page

Title: *The Mindset of Weight Loss: Unlocking Mental Habits for Lasting Change*

Author: Anthony Ezigbo

**Copyright © 2024 by Anthony Ezigbo*

All rights reserved.

Publisher:

Anthony Ezigbo

Owerri, Imo, Nigeria. 460104

anthonyezigbo@yahoo.com

This is a work of nonfiction. While every effort has been made to ensure that the information contained in this book is accurate, the author and publisher assume no responsibility for errors or omissions. The advice and strategies contained herein may not be suitable for your situation. You should consult with a professional where appropriate.

Disclaimer:

The information provided in this book is for educational and informational purposes only. It is not intended as a substitute for professional medical advice, diagnosis, or treatment. Always seek the advice of your physician or other qualified health providers with any questions you may have regarding a medical condition. The author is not responsible for any actions taken by the reader as a result of the information provided in this book.

Amazon Kindle Direct Publishing Edition
First Edition: September, 2024

Dedication

To everyone who has ever struggled with the weight of their mind as much as their body.

This book is for those seeking lasting change, for those ready to break free from limiting beliefs, and for those committed to transforming not only their physical selves but their inner world as well.

May you find the strength, clarity, and courage to unlock your full potential and live a life of balance, health, and self-love.

Here's to your journey—may it be as rewarding as your destination.

Table of Contents

Foreword

A Journey to Sustainable Weight Loss Through Mindset

We live in a world where weight loss is often reduced to quick fixes, fad diets, and fleeting moments of motivation. Too often, we're told that losing weight is just a matter of willpower or following the latest trending plan. But, as anyone who has tried—and struggled—to lose weight knows, there is much more to the story. It's not just about what we eat, how much we exercise, or what diet we follow. It's about the mindset we bring to the entire process.

This book you hold in your hands is a powerful reminder that sustainable weight loss isn't about restriction, deprivation, or force. It's about transformation—from the inside out. It's about reprogramming the way you think about food, exercise, and most importantly, yourself. **Sustainable weight loss is not a sprint, it's a lifelong journey**—and the path to lasting change begins in the mind.

One of the key messages of this book is that **weight loss isn't simply about shedding pounds**; it's about **shedding limiting beliefs**, negative habits, and unhealthy mental patterns that keep you stuck in a cycle of failure and frustration. You'll learn that the way you talk to yourself, the habits you build, and the environment you create are just as important—if not more so—than the number on the scale.

Throughout the chapters, you'll be guided through strategies that go far beyond willpower. You'll discover why **discipline triumphs over willpower** and how cultivating daily habits—

small, sustainable changes—can transform not just your body, but your entire life. This book emphasizes the importance of consistency and routine, showing you how to build new habits that stick by leveraging the science of habit formation. Whether it's through **habit stacking**, creating a supportive environment, or using visualization techniques, you will find practical tools to ensure that you're building a lifestyle, not just following a diet.

You'll also be introduced to the idea that weight loss is deeply intertwined with your emotional and mental well-being. **Mindful eating**, understanding emotional triggers, and learning to manage stress without turning to food are all integral parts of this journey. In fact, **the mind-body connection** is a key theme throughout the book—helping you to recognize that true transformation happens when you begin to care for both your mental and physical health in tandem. Whether it's through mindful eating, meditation, or exercise as a tool for stress relief, this book shows how weight loss and mental clarity go hand in hand.

And yet, there is no illusion here that the road is easy. Weight loss comes with challenges—setbacks, plateaus, and moments of discouragement. But this book equips you with the mental tools to **overcome obstacles, bounce back from failures, and build resilience**. It's not about perfection—it's about progress. **It's about turning setbacks into comebacks** and continuing to move forward even when the journey feels difficult.

This book also encourages you to break free from the isolation that often comes with weight loss. You'll learn how to create a **supportive community** of like-minded individuals, accountability partners, and even professionals who can help you stay on track. You don't have to go it alone. Building a positive, empowering network is essential for long-term success, and this book shows you how to do just that.

But perhaps most importantly, this book reminds you that **your relationship with food can be one of balance, joy, and freedom**. It's not about rigid rules or punishing yourself with restriction. Instead, you'll learn how to develop a healthy, intuitive relationship with food—one that allows you to enjoy what you eat without guilt or anxiety. With strategies like the **80/20 rule** and **intuitive eating**, you'll begin to trust your body's cues and make choices that nourish both your body and soul.

As you turn these pages, you're not just embarking on a journey to lose weight—you're embarking on a journey to change your mindset, your habits, and your relationship with yourself. The tools and insights in this book will help you build a foundation of mental strength and resilience that will carry you far beyond weight loss. You'll find the confidence to not only reach your goals but to maintain your success and continue growing long after the weight is gone.

This book is your companion for the road ahead. It's a roadmap for navigating the challenges, celebrating the victories, and embracing the journey to a healthier, more empowered you. Whether you're just beginning your weight loss journey or you're looking for a way to sustain the progress you've already made, this book offers the wisdom, practical tools, and encouragement you need.

As you begin this journey, remember: **You are capable of change. You are worthy of success. And you have everything you need within you to create the life you desire.**

Here's to your transformation, your success, and your healthiest, happiest self. The journey begins now.

Introduction

The Power of Mindset in Weight Loss

When it comes to weight loss, the first things that come to mind are diet plans, workout routines, and calorie counting. However, while these elements are essential, they often overshadow an equally, if not more critical, component of the weight loss journey: mindset. A successful weight loss transformation is as much about mental strength, emotional resilience, and habit change as it is about physical activity and nutrition. In fact, one could argue that without the right mindset, lasting weight loss is almost impossible to achieve.

Importance of Mindset in Weight Loss Success

Mindset is the foundation on which everything else in a weight loss journey rests. It's the key to staying motivated, overcoming obstacles, and maintaining the discipline required to make real and lasting changes. In the world of weight loss, your mindset is what keeps you going when the excitement of starting something new wears off, when the scale isn't moving as quickly as you'd like, or when temptation calls at the end of a long day.

Why is mindset so crucial in the weight loss process? The answer lies in how our thoughts, beliefs, and attitudes shape our actions. People who have a fixed mindset tend to believe their abilities are set in stone. They often feel powerless to change their circumstances and may give up when faced with difficulties. On the other hand, those with a growth mindset see challenges as opportunities to learn and grow. They understand that failure is a part of the journey and that perseverance is key to achieving their goals.

When you adopt a growth mindset in weight loss, you no longer view setbacks as reasons to quit. Instead, you learn to see them as valuable feedback, signals of what's not working, and opportunities to adjust your approach. This shift in thinking helps you stay committed to the process, even when progress is slow or when you encounter difficulties.

A crucial aspect of mindset in weight loss is self-compassion. Too often, people approach weight loss with a sense of harsh discipline, using negative self-talk to "motivate" themselves. Phrases like "I'll never lose weight" or "I'm just not disciplined enough" are common and can sabotage progress. By contrast, a mindset rooted in self-compassion allows for grace and patience. It acknowledges that setbacks are normal and encourages you to treat yourself kindly when things don't go perfectly.

The Role of Habits and Psychology in Achieving Lasting Change

While the idea of willpower often dominates conversations about weight loss, research shows that lasting change comes not from sheer force of will but from building sustainable habits. Habits are powerful because they allow us to perform actions without thinking. Once a behavior becomes habitual, it no longer requires the same level of mental energy or discipline. This is why people who have successfully lost weight and kept it off often credit not their willpower, but the new habits they've formed.

The role of psychology in habit formation is significant. At its core, habit formation is about creating new neural pathways in the brain. The more we repeat a behavior, the more ingrained it becomes in our daily routine. However, this process takes time, which is why quick fixes or fad diets rarely lead to lasting results. For sustainable weight loss, we need to focus on building small, positive habits that can be maintained in the long run.

Understanding the psychology of habits also means recognizing the role of triggers and rewards. Every habit has a cue that initiates the behavior, followed by the behavior itself, and then a reward that reinforces it. For example, if you tend to reach for junk food when you're stressed, the cue might be the feeling of stress, the behavior is eating, and the reward is the temporary relief from that stress. To change this habit, you need to find a different behavior (such as going for a walk or practicing deep breathing) that provides a similar reward. This process requires self-awareness and a willingness to experiment with different strategies until you find what works for you.

One of the biggest psychological barriers to weight loss is the "all-or-nothing" mentality. This mindset leads people to believe that if they make one mistake, their entire day—or even their entire effort—is ruined. For instance, eating an unplanned slice of cake at a party might make someone feel like they've failed, leading them to abandon their diet for the rest of the day. But lasting change comes from understanding that perfection is not the goal. In fact, those who succeed in weight loss are often those who can quickly bounce back from small missteps. They understand that one slip-up doesn't define their entire journey and that each day is an opportunity to start fresh.

Overview of the Book: What Readers Will Learn

This book, *The Mindset of Weight Loss: Unlocking Mental Habits for Lasting Change*, is designed to equip you with the psychological tools and mental strategies you need to achieve your weight loss goals and maintain them for life. Throughout the following chapters, we will explore the intricate relationship between mindset, habits, and sustainable weight loss, and how you can leverage the power of your mind to create lasting, meaningful change in your life.

The journey begins by delving deeper into how our thoughts, beliefs, and attitudes influence our behaviors, particularly when it comes to weight loss. We'll look at common mental roadblocks that prevent people from reaching their goals, such as self-sabotage, fear of failure, and emotional eating. You'll learn to identify these patterns in your own life and develop strategies to overcome them.

Next, we'll focus on the science of habits. You'll discover how to break unhealthy patterns and replace them with new, positive ones. This process will require patience and consistency, but by following the techniques outlined in this book, you'll be able to create habits that support your weight loss journey and your overall well-being. We'll also explore the concept of "keystone habits"—those small changes that can have a ripple effect across multiple areas of your life—and how they can be applied to weight loss.

Additionally, we'll address the emotional side of weight loss. Many people struggle with emotional eating, using food as a way to cope with stress, sadness, or even boredom. This book will help you understand the root causes of emotional eating and provide you with practical tools to manage your emotions in a healthier way, without relying on food for comfort.

Another critical aspect of the book will be the importance of goal-setting. Setting realistic, achievable goals is a crucial part of any weight loss journey, but equally important is understanding the "why" behind your goals. We'll guide you through the process of identifying your deeper motivations for wanting to lose weight and help you stay focused on those reasons, even when the going gets tough.

Throughout the book, you'll also find practical exercises and reflective prompts to help you apply what you're learning to your own life. This is not just a book to read—it's a book to interact with, to use as a tool for real change. Each chapter builds on the last, providing you with a step-by-step framework for transforming your mindset, building healthy habits, and achieving lasting weight loss.

By the end of this book, you'll have a deep understanding of how your mind works in relation to weight loss and how you can harness its power to create the life you want. You'll walk away with actionable strategies for building a positive, resilient mindset, breaking free from destructive patterns, and creating lasting change. Most importantly, you'll learn that the secret to successful weight loss lies not in following a rigid diet plan, but in unlocking the potential of your mind.

In this journey, you will discover that true weight loss success isn't about reaching a number on the scale; it's about transforming your relationship with food, with your body, and with yourself. With the right mindset, anything is possible.

25

Chapter 1
Understanding the Weight Loss Mindset

The Difference Between Short-Term and Long-Term Weight Loss

When most people think about weight loss, their immediate goal is to see the number on the scale drop. This is often achieved through quick-fix diets, extreme calorie restriction, or rigorous exercise regimens. While these methods may lead to short-term results, they often fail to create lasting change. The reason behind this lies not just in the physical mechanisms of the body, but in the mindset driving these actions. Understanding the difference between short-term and long-term weight loss is crucial for anyone serious about achieving sustainable results.

Short-term weight loss is often the product of a temporary surge of motivation. You may be inspired by a special event, a vacation, or dissatisfaction with how you look and feel. In these instances, the urgency to shed pounds quickly overrides other considerations. The focus is on fast results, and this typically leads people to adopt unsustainable habits. Popular crash diets, detoxes, or extreme exercise programs can certainly lead to visible changes, but because they don't address the root of why weight was gained in the first place, the results are often fleeting.

The problem with short-term weight loss is that it's driven by external goals—looking good for a wedding, a reunion, or summer. Once the goal is achieved, or when motivation fades, old habits return, and the weight comes back, sometimes even more than before. This creates a yo-yo effect, where individuals cycle between losing and gaining weight, often damaging their metabolism and self-esteem in the process.

Long-term weight loss, on the other hand, is about more than just shedding pounds; it's about creating a healthy, balanced lifestyle that you can maintain indefinitely. This approach focuses not just on the physical aspects of losing weight but also on the mental, emotional, and behavioral changes required to sustain those results. The key difference is the mindset: instead of focusing on a short-term number on the scale, the focus shifts to developing sustainable habits that promote overall well-being.

Long-term weight loss involves learning to approach food, exercise, and self-care in a balanced, flexible manner. It's about adopting a growth mindset, where you recognize that success comes from consistency and small, incremental improvements. This approach is less about perfection and more about progress. It acknowledges that setbacks will happen but emphasizes resilience, self-compassion, and a commitment to getting back on track.

The primary difference between short-term and long-term weight loss comes down to this: short-term weight loss is reactive and driven by immediate gratification, whereas long-term weight loss is proactive, focusing on sustainable lifestyle changes and self-awareness. Achieving long-term weight loss requires shifting your mindset from quick fixes to lifelong habits, and that begins with understanding why dieting alone doesn't work.

Why Dieting Alone Doesn't Work: A Mental Perspective

The weight loss industry is flooded with countless diets promising quick results. From low-carb to low-fat, from keto to intermittent fasting, there's no shortage of methods that claim to be the ultimate solution. While some diets may be effective in the short term, the majority of people find that dieting alone doesn't lead to lasting results. In fact, studies have shown that most people regain the weight they lose on diets within a year. Why is that?

The answer lies in how dieting affects your mindset and relationship with food. When you start a diet, you're often adopting a restrictive mindset. You create a set of rules around what you can and cannot eat, and while this can work in the short term, it's rarely sustainable over the long term. Diets operate on the principle of deprivation, which not only makes you feel like you're missing out but also leads to increased cravings for the very foods you're trying to avoid.

Psychologically, this creates a vicious cycle: you restrict, which leads to cravings, which often leads to a "binge," followed by guilt and shame. This, in turn, often leads to more restrictive behavior, starting the cycle all over again. Over time, this pattern can lead to disordered eating, a poor relationship with food, and a damaging sense of failure when the diet inevitably doesn't work.

Dieting also creates an external locus of control. When you're following a diet, you're often relying on external rules—whether that's calorie counting, macronutrient ratios, or eating within certain windows of time—to guide your behavior. This means that your sense of success or failure is tied to how well you adhere to these external guidelines. But when life inevitably gets in the way—whether through a social event, travel, or just a stressful day at work—those rules can become hard to follow. Without a deeper understanding of your internal motivations and the psychology behind your food choices, it's easy to fall off track and abandon the diet altogether.

What dieting misses is the need for internal transformation. True, lasting weight loss requires addressing the underlying reasons why you overeat or make unhealthy choices. Emotional eating, stress, boredom, and social pressures all play a significant role in weight gain, and no diet plan can address these psychological triggers. Without a shift in mindset and behavior, any progress made on a diet is likely to be temporary.

Shifting from a "Diet" Mentality to a "Lifestyle" Mentality

So, if dieting alone doesn't work, what's the alternative? The answer lies in shifting from a "diet" mentality to a "lifestyle" mentality. A lifestyle mentality is about creating healthy habits that you can maintain for the rest of your life, rather than following a temporary set of rules to achieve a short-term goal. This shift is critical for long-term weight loss success because it focuses on building a foundation of sustainable behaviors rather than relying on willpower and restriction.

To make this shift, it's important to change the way you think about food and exercise. Instead of viewing certain foods as "good" or "bad," or exercise as a punishment for overeating, you begin to see them as tools for nourishing and supporting your body. This shift allows you to approach weight loss from a place of self-care rather than self-deprivation.

Here are a few key mindset shifts that can help you transition from a diet mentality to a lifestyle mentality:

1. **Focus on Progress, Not Perfection**
   One of the biggest traps of the diet mentality is the belief that you need to follow your plan perfectly in order to be successful. If you slip up, it's easy to feel like you've failed and abandon your efforts altogether. In a lifestyle mentality, however, you understand that progress is more important than perfection. You allow yourself room for flexibility and understand that one slip-up doesn't define your entire journey. This shift in thinking helps reduce feelings of guilt and shame and allows you to bounce back more quickly from setbacks.

2. **Listen to Your Body**

   Diets often encourage you to ignore your body's natural hunger and fullness cues in favor of following rigid rules about what and when to eat. This can lead to overeating, bingeing, or a disconnection from your body's needs. In contrast, a lifestyle mentality encourages you to tune into your body's signals and eat in a way that feels satisfying and nourishing. This approach, often referred to as intuitive eating, helps you develop a healthier relationship with food and reduces the likelihood of overeating or emotional eating.

3. **Emphasize Long-Term Health Over Short-Term Weight Loss**

   In a diet mentality, the focus is often on achieving quick results, regardless of the impact on your overall health. Extreme calorie restriction, for example, can lead to rapid weight loss but can also slow down your metabolism, increase your stress levels, and leave you feeling fatigued and irritable. A lifestyle mentality, on the other hand, emphasizes long-term health and well-being. Instead of focusing solely on the scale, you start to prioritize how you feel—your energy levels, your mental clarity, your mood, and your overall quality of life.

4. **Practice Self-Compassion**

One of the hallmarks of the diet mentality is harsh self-criticism. If you slip up or don't see immediate results, it's easy to fall into a pattern of negative self-talk. But this only serves to sabotage your efforts in the long run. A lifestyle mentality, by contrast, encourages self-compassion. You treat yourself with kindness and understanding, recognizing that weight loss is a journey, not a race. By practicing self-compassion, you build resilience and are more likely to stay committed to your goals, even when progress is slow.

5. **Make Sustainable Changes**

   Diets are often unsustainable because they ask you to make drastic changes that are difficult to maintain over time. A lifestyle mentality, on the other hand, focuses on making small, sustainable changes that you can stick with in the long term. This might mean gradually increasing your intake of vegetables, finding forms of exercise that you enjoy, or learning new ways to manage stress. The key is to make changes that fit into your life, rather than trying to overhaul your entire routine overnight.

Case Studies: How Mindset Shifts Led to Successful Weight Loss

To illustrate the power of mindset in weight loss, let's explore a few real-life case studies of individuals who experienced significant transformations by shifting their mindset.

Case Study 1: Sarah's Shift from All-or-Nothing Thinking

Sarah had been struggling with her weight for years, cycling between extreme diets and periods of overeating. Her all-or-nothing mentality kept her stuck in a cycle of starting and abandoning diets. After learning about the importance of mindset, Sarah decided to take a different approach. She focused on progress, not perfection, and allowed herself to enjoy occasional treats without feeling guilty. This mindset shift helped her stay consistent with her healthy habits, and over the course of a year, she lost 40 pounds and maintained her new weight.

Case Study 2: James' Journey to Mindful Eating

James was an emotional eater, turning to food for comfort during times of stress. He had tried numerous diets, but they never addressed the root of his overeating. After working with a coach to develop a healthier mindset, James began practicing mindful eating. He learned to listen to his body's hunger and fullness cues and became more aware of the emotional triggers that led to overeating. By shifting his mindset from deprivation to mindfulness, James not only lost 30 pounds but also developed a healthier relationship with food.

Case Study 3: Maria's Focus on Health, Not Just Weight

Maria had always focused on the scale as the primary measure of her success. But after years of yo-yo dieting, she realized that her obsession with weight loss was taking a toll on her mental and physical health. Maria decided to shift her focus to overall well-being. She began prioritizing sleep, stress management, and self-care, and as a result, her energy levels improved, and she felt more balanced. Over time, she lost 25 pounds, but more importantly, she felt healthier and happier than she had in years.

These case studies highlight the transformative power of a mindset shift. By moving away from a diet mentality and embracing a lifestyle approach, these individuals were able to achieve lasting weight loss and improve their overall well-being.

Understanding the weight loss mindset is crucial for achieving long-term success. While short-term diets may provide quick results, they often fail to address the deeper psychological factors that contribute to weight gain. By shifting from a diet mentality to a lifestyle mentality, you can create sustainable habits that promote lasting health and well-being. This shift requires focusing on progress rather than perfection, listening to your body, emphasizing long-term health over short-term weight loss, practicing self-compassion, and making sustainable changes. With the right mindset, weight loss becomes not just about achieving a number on the scale but about creating a healthier, more fulfilling life.

Chapter 2

Breaking Free from Limiting Beliefs

Weight loss is not just about what you eat or how much you exercise. A significant part of the journey lies in your mind—particularly in your beliefs about yourself, your abilities, and your potential. Limiting beliefs can quietly sabotage your efforts and prevent you from reaching your goals, no matter how dedicated you are to physical changes. These beliefs often take the form of negative self-talk, unhelpful mental habits, and an "all-or-nothing" mentality. In this chapter, we will explore how to identify and break free from these limiting beliefs, and provide practical tools and exercises to help you transform them into empowering, positive thoughts.

Common Self-Limiting Beliefs that Sabotage Weight Loss Efforts

Limiting beliefs are assumptions or convictions that hold you back from achieving your true potential. When it comes to weight loss, these beliefs can often become deeply ingrained, shaping how you think, act, and feel about yourself. Let's examine some of the most common limiting beliefs that can sabotage your weight loss efforts.

1. **"I've always been overweight; it's just who I am."**

   This belief can trap you in a cycle of hopelessness. If you believe that being overweight is an unchangeable part of your identity, you may feel powerless to make changes, even when you're motivated. The truth is, your past does not define your future. Your body is capable of transformation when you commit to lasting change and address the habits and thoughts that have kept you stuck.

2. **"I don't deserve to be healthy and happy."**

Many people struggle with feelings of unworthiness when it comes to weight loss. This belief may stem from past failures, low self-esteem, or a history of criticism. When you feel like you don't deserve to look and feel your best, it's easy to self-sabotage by giving up or making unhealthy choices. Remember, everyone deserves health, happiness, and self-love.

3. **"I'll never be able to lose weight—it's too hard."**

This limiting belief is rooted in fear of

failure. If you've tried to lose weight before and haven't succeeded, it's natural to feel like it's an impossible task. However, weight loss isn't about achieving perfection; it's about consistency and persistence. Believing in your ability to succeed is the first step toward achieving your goals.

4. **"I've tried everything, and nothing works for me."**

Many people feel discouraged after trying multiple diets or exercise routines without long-term success. This belief can lead to feelings of frustration and resignation. The reality is, weight loss is not a one-size-fits-all process. What works for someone else may not work for you, and it may take time to find the right approach. But that doesn't mean success is out of reach—it simply means you need to find a plan that suits your unique needs and mindset.

5. **"If I can't do it perfectly, it's not worth trying."**

Perfectionism is a common roadblock to weight loss. This belief sets impossibly high standards, where any slip-up or deviation from the plan feels like failure. The truth is, progress is made in the small, imperfect steps you take every day. Embracing imperfection and learning from setbacks is essential for long-term success.

6. **"I don't have the time, energy, or resources to lose weight."**

This belief stems from a scarcity mindset, where you feel like you lack the necessary tools or circumstances to achieve your goals. While it's true that life can be busy and challenging, there's always a way to prioritize your health, whether it's by setting small, manageable goals or finding creative ways to incorporate healthier habits into your routine.

Recognizing these limiting beliefs is the first step toward freeing yourself from them. Once you understand the thoughts that are holding you back, you can begin to challenge and reframe them into more empowering beliefs.

How to Identify Negative Self-Talk and Reframe It

Negative self-talk is one of the most insidious ways that limiting beliefs manifest. It's the inner dialogue that tells you that you're not good enough, that you'll never succeed, or that you're destined to fail. The problem with negative self-talk is that it often happens so automatically that you don't even realize it's there. Yet, these thoughts can have a powerful impact on your behavior and your progress.

The first step in combating negative self-talk is awareness. You need to tune into your internal dialogue and notice the patterns in your thinking. Here are some ways to identify negative self-talk:

1. **Pay attention to how you talk to yourself when you make a mistake.** When you skip a workout or eat something off-plan, what's your immediate response? Do you think, "I always mess up" or "I'm such a failure"? These are examples of negative self-talk. Instead, try to recognize the mistake without judging yourself harshly. You can say, "I missed a workout today, but I'll make sure to get back on track tomorrow."

2. **Look for "all-or-nothing" language.**
   Words like "always," "never," and "can't" are often signs of limiting beliefs. For example, saying "I can't stick to any diet" or "I never succeed" reinforces a negative narrative about your abilities. Challenge these thoughts by replacing absolute statements with more flexible language, such as, "I've struggled in the past, but I'm learning how to be more consistent."

3. **Notice how you speak about your body.**
   Body image is a major source of negative self-talk for many people. If you frequently catch yourself thinking, "I hate my body" or "I'll never look good," it's time to reframe those thoughts. Start by acknowledging your body's strengths and capabilities. Instead of focusing on what you don't

like, appreciate what your body can do, such as, "My body is strong and capable of change."

Once you've identified your negative self-talk, the next step is to reframe it into more positive, empowering statements. This doesn't mean ignoring challenges or pretending everything is perfect, but it does mean shifting your focus from self-criticism to self-compassion. Here are some examples of how to reframe common negative thoughts:

- **Negative Thought**: "I'll never be able to lose this weight."
  Reframed Thought: "Losing weight is challenging, but I can take it one step at a time and make progress."
- **Negative Thought**: "I messed up today, so there's no point in trying anymore."
  Reframed Thought: "One mistake

doesn't define my journey. I can learn from it and get back on track."

- **Negative Thought**: "I don't deserve to feel good about myself."
  Reframed Thought: "I am worthy of health and happiness, and I'm taking steps to improve my well-being."
- **Negative Thought**: "If I can't do it perfectly, I shouldn't even try."
  Reframed Thought: "Progress is made through effort, not perfection. Every small step counts."

By consistently reframing your negative thoughts, you'll begin to change the narrative you have about yourself and your abilities. This process takes time and practice, but it's an essential part of breaking free from limiting beliefs.

Overcoming the "All-or-Nothing" Mentality

The "all-or-nothing" mentality is one of the most common limiting beliefs that can hinder your weight loss journey. It's the belief that if you're not doing everything perfectly, then your efforts don't count at all. This mentality often leads to cycles of extreme restriction followed by periods of overeating or giving up entirely. For example, if you eat one "unhealthy" meal, you might think, "Well, I've already blown it, so I might as well eat whatever I want for the rest of the day."

The "all-or-nothing" mentality is harmful because it sets unrealistic expectations and encourages black-and-white thinking. It prevents you from seeing the value in small, consistent efforts and leads to a sense of failure whenever you deviate from your plan.

To overcome this mentality, it's important to embrace the concept of **balance** and **progress over perfection**. Here are some practical steps to help you break free from the "all-or-nothing" mindset:

1. **Set Realistic Expectations**

   Instead of aiming for perfection, focus on making small, manageable changes that you can sustain over time. For example, rather than trying to overhaul your entire diet in one week, start by adding more vegetables to your meals or cutting back on sugary snacks. These small changes may not feel as dramatic as a restrictive diet, but they are more likely to lead to lasting results.

   "Success is the sum of small efforts, repeated day in and day out." – Robert Collier

2. **Allow for Flexibility**

   Life is unpredictable, and there will be times when you can't stick to your plan perfectly—and that's okay. Flexibility is key to long-term success. Instead of feeling guilty or giving up when you go off-plan, remind yourself that one meal, one workout, or one day does not define your entire journey. You can always make a positive choice in the next moment.

3. **Celebrate Small Wins**

   Recognize and celebrate your progress, no matter how small. Did you drink more water today? Did you go for a walk when you didn't feel like it? These small wins add up and contribute to your overall success. By focusing on what you're doing right, rather than what you think you're doing wrong, you'll stay motivated and positive.

4. **Practice Self-Compassion**

   Be kind to yourself when things don't go as planned. Weight loss is a journey, and there will be ups and downs along the way. Instead of criticizing yourself for a mistake, practice self-compassion by acknowledging that everyone struggles at times. Use setbacks as learning opportunities rather than reasons to quit.

   "You are allowed to be both a masterpiece and a work in progress simultaneously." – Sophia Bush

5. **Adopt a Growth Mindset**

   A growth mindset is the belief that your abilities and intelligence can be developed through effort and learning. When you adopt a growth mindset, you view challenges and setbacks as opportunities for growth rather than signs of failure. This mindset is essential for overcoming the "all-or-nothing" mentality because it encourages resilience and perseverance.

"Success is not final; failure is not fatal: It is the courage to continue that counts." – Winston Churchill

Practical Exercises for Transforming Limiting Beliefs into Empowering Ones

To break free from limiting beliefs, it's essential to take practical steps to rewire your thinking. Here are some exercises you can use to transform your limiting beliefs into empowering ones:

1. **Identify Your Limiting Beliefs**
   Take a few moments to reflect on the

beliefs you hold about weight loss, your abilities, and your potential for success. Write down any negative or limiting thoughts that come to mind. For example, you might write, "I've always struggled with my weight, so I'll never be able to lose it."

2. **Challenge Your Beliefs**

   Once you've identified your limiting beliefs, ask yourself: Are these beliefs based on facts, or are they just assumptions? What evidence do I have to support or refute this belief? For example, if your belief is "I'll never lose weight," challenge that by asking, "Is it really true that I can't lose weight, or is it possible that I haven't found the right approach yet?"

3. **Create Empowering Affirmations**

   For each limiting belief, create a positive affirmation that counters it. For example, if your limiting belief is "I don't deserve to be healthy," your affirmation might be "I deserve to feel good in my body and live a healthy, vibrant life." Repeat these affirmations to yourself daily, especially when you notice negative thoughts creeping in.

4. **Visualization**

Visualization is a powerful tool for shifting your mindset. Take a few minutes each day to visualize yourself achieving your weight loss goals. Imagine how it will feel to reach your goal weight, how your body will feel, and how your life will change. The more vividly you can imagine your success, the more motivated you'll feel to take the necessary actions.

"What the mind can conceive and believe, it can achieve." – Napoleon Hill

5. **Journaling**

Journaling is a great way to process your thoughts and emotions around weight loss. Each day, write about your progress, your challenges, and any limiting beliefs that come up. Use this time to reflect on how you can reframe negative thoughts and focus on the positive changes you're making.

Breaking free from limiting beliefs is a crucial part of any weight loss journey. By identifying and challenging these beliefs, reframing negative self-talk, overcoming the "all-or-nothing" mentality, and practicing self-compassion, you can create a mindset that supports lasting success. Remember, weight loss is not just about changing your body—it's about transforming your mind and believing in your ability to achieve your goals. With the right mindset, anything is possible.

Chapter 3

The Role of Emotional Eating

Weight loss is as much about managing emotions as it is about food choices and exercise routines. Emotional eating, the act of using food to cope with feelings rather than satisfy physical hunger, can be one of the biggest obstacles to achieving lasting weight loss. It is deeply rooted in our psychology and can often derail even the best-laid plans for a healthy lifestyle. To truly succeed in your weight loss journey, it is crucial to understand the role of emotions in your eating habits, recognize emotional triggers, and develop strategies to cope with these feelings in healthier ways.

In this chapter, we will explore emotional eating in depth, from identifying emotional triggers to differentiating between physical and emotional hunger. You will also learn practical strategies to address stress, boredom, and other emotional triggers, as well as mindful eating techniques to stay present during meals. Lastly, we will look at personal stories of individuals who have overcome emotional eating, offering real-life inspiration for how you can do the same.

Understanding Emotional Triggers for Overeating

Emotional eating is a learned behavior. From childhood, many of us are conditioned to associate food with comfort, reward, or even distraction. Whether it's reaching for a tub of ice cream after a bad day or mindlessly snacking while watching TV to avoid feelings of boredom or stress, emotional eating can become a go-to coping mechanism.

Some common emotional triggers for overeating include:

1. **Stress**

   Stress is one of the most prevalent triggers for emotional eating. When we're stressed, our bodies release cortisol, a hormone that can increase cravings for high-fat, high-sugar foods. Eating these "comfort" foods temporarily soothes the discomfort of stress, but it also reinforces the habit of turning to food for emotional relief.

2. **Boredom**

   Many people eat out of boredom, simply because they're not engaged in anything else. Food becomes a way to fill the void, offering distraction and momentary satisfaction. However, this type of eating rarely comes from physical hunger, and it can lead to overeating without realizing it.

3. **Loneliness**

Emotional eating is often a response to loneliness. Food can serve as a substitute for connection and companionship, providing comfort in the absence of social support. The act of eating may momentarily relieve feelings of isolation, but it doesn't address the root cause of loneliness.

4. **Sadness or Depression**

For some, food becomes a way to numb difficult emotions such as sadness or depression. Emotional eaters may turn to food in an attempt to fill an emotional void or to experience a fleeting sense of pleasure that temporarily lifts their mood.

5. **Celebration or Reward**

Emotional eating doesn't always stem from negative emotions. Many people associate food with positive emotions, such as celebration or reward. For example, after completing a difficult task or reaching a milestone, you might feel like you "deserve" to indulge. While there's nothing wrong with enjoying food as part of a celebration, it can become problematic when it turns into a frequent way to reward yourself for everyday achievements.

Understanding your emotional triggers is the first step toward breaking the cycle of emotional eating. Once you can identify what emotions drive your eating behavior, you can start developing healthier ways to cope with those feelings.

How to Differentiate Between Physical Hunger and Emotional Hunger

One of the biggest challenges in overcoming emotional eating is learning how to distinguish between physical hunger and emotional hunger. While physical hunger is your body's natural signal that it needs fuel, emotional hunger is driven by feelings and is not connected to your body's energy needs.

Here are some key differences between physical and emotional hunger:

1. **Physical Hunger**
   - Develops gradually
   - Can be satisfied with a variety of foods
   - Leads to feelings of satisfaction and fullness after eating

- o You're aware of when you last ate and can recognize when it's time for your next meal
- o You're willing to wait for food or make a healthy choice

2. **Emotional Hunger**

- o Comes on suddenly and feels urgent
- o Craves specific comfort foods (often high in sugar, fat, or carbs)
- o Doesn't lead to satisfaction, often leaving you feeling guilty or unfulfilled
- o Is unrelated to when you last ate, and you might not even feel physically hungry
- o Makes you want to eat immediately, regardless of what's available

A helpful way to differentiate between the two is to pause before eating and ask yourself, "Am I truly hungry, or am I trying to soothe an emotion?" By creating a moment of awareness, you can start to become more mindful of your eating habits and make more intentional choices.

Practical Strategies to Deal with Stress, Boredom, and Emotional Triggers

Once you've identified the emotional triggers that lead to overeating, the next step is to develop healthier coping mechanisms. While it may not be realistic to eliminate stress, boredom, or loneliness from your life, you can control how you respond to these emotions. Here are some practical strategies to deal with common emotional triggers.

1. Managing Stress Without Food

Since stress is such a common trigger for emotional eating, it's important to find alternative ways to cope with it. Some effective stress-relief techniques include:

- **Exercise**: Physical activity is a great way to reduce stress and boost your mood. Exercise releases endorphins, the body's natural stress relievers, and can help distract you from stressful thoughts. Whether it's a brisk walk, yoga, or a workout at the gym, find an activity that you enjoy and can turn to when stress levels rise.

- **Meditation or Deep Breathing**: Mindfulness meditation or deep breathing exercises can help you stay grounded and reduce anxiety. Taking just a few minutes to focus on your breath can calm your nervous system and reduce the urge to eat emotionally.

- **Journaling**: Writing about your feelings can be a powerful way to process emotions without turning to food. When you're feeling stressed or overwhelmed, take a few minutes to jot down what's on your mind. This can help you identify the source of your stress and provide a sense of relief.

- **Progressive Muscle Relaxation**: This technique involves tensing and relaxing different muscle groups in your body to reduce physical tension. It's an effective way to manage stress and can be done in just a few minutes.

2. Addressing Boredom

To combat boredom eating, it's important to find alternative activities that engage your mind and body. Some ideas include:

- **Engage in a Hobby**: Instead of reaching for snacks when you're bored, find a hobby or activity that you enjoy, such as reading, knitting, painting, or playing a musical instrument. These activities provide a mental challenge and can keep you occupied without food.

- **Go for a Walk**: Getting outside and moving your body is a great way to break up boredom. A change of scenery can refresh your mind and distract you from the urge to eat.

- **Learn Something New**: Challenge yourself by learning a new skill, such as cooking a healthy recipe, picking up a language, or taking an online course. Engaging your mind in learning can reduce the temptation to eat out of boredom.

3. Dealing with Loneliness

If loneliness is a trigger for emotional eating, it's important to focus on building meaningful connections and finding ways to fill your emotional needs. Some ways to combat loneliness include:

- **Reach Out to Friends or Family**: When you're feeling lonely, call or text a friend or family member. Even a brief conversation can help lift your spirits and reduce the desire to eat emotionally.
- **Join a Support Group**: Connecting with others who are going through similar experiences can provide emotional support and reduce feelings of isolation. Look for local or online support groups focused on weight loss, emotional eating, or mental health.
- **Volunteer or Get Involved in Your Community**: Volunteering is a great

way to connect with others and make a positive impact. It can also give you a sense of purpose and reduce feelings of loneliness.

4. Coping with Sadness or Depression

When sadness or depression triggers emotional eating, it's important to address the underlying emotions. Some strategies include:

- **Seek Professional Help**: If you're struggling with depression, talking to a therapist or counselor can help you work through your emotions and develop healthier coping mechanisms.

- **Practice Self-Care**: Taking care of yourself emotionally and physically can improve your mood and reduce the urge to eat emotionally. Self-care can include activities such as taking a bath, getting a massage, or spending time in nature.

- **Express Your Emotions**: Rather than bottling up your emotions, find healthy ways to express them. This could include talking to a trusted friend, writing in a journal, or engaging in creative outlets like art or music.

Mindful Eating: Techniques to Stay Present During Meals

Mindful eating is a powerful tool for overcoming emotional eating. It involves being fully present during your meals, paying attention to the experience of eating without judgment, and listening to your body's hunger and fullness cues.

Here are some mindful eating techniques to help you stay present during meals:

1. **Eat Slowly**
   One of the best ways to practice mindful

eating is to slow down. Eating slowly allows you to savor each bite and tune in to your body's signals of hunger and fullness. It also gives your brain time to register when you're full, which can prevent overeating.

2. **Eliminate Distractions**

When you eat in front of the TV, at your desk, or while scrolling through your phone, it's easy to lose track of how much you're eating. To practice mindful eating, eliminate distractions and focus solely on your meal. This helps you become more aware of what you're eating and how much.

3. **Chew Thoroughly**

Chewing your food thoroughly not only aids digestion but also helps you eat more mindfully. By chewing each bite slowly and thoroughly, you can fully experience the taste, texture, and aroma of your food.

4. **Listen to Your Body**

   Pay attention to your body's hunger and fullness cues. Eat when you're physically hungry, and stop when you're comfortably full. This helps you avoid emotional eating and ensures that you're eating to nourish your body rather than to satisfy emotional needs.

5. **Engage Your Senses**

   Mindful eating involves engaging all of your senses in the eating experience. Notice the colors, smells, textures, and flavors of your food. By bringing awareness to the sensory aspects of eating, you can become more present and enjoy your meals more fully.

Personal Stories: Overcoming Emotional Eating

Hearing personal stories of individuals who have successfully overcome emotional eating can be a source of inspiration and motivation. These stories demonstrate that change is possible, even when emotional eating feels like an insurmountable challenge.

Story 1: Sarah's Journey

Sarah had struggled with emotional eating for years, particularly during stressful periods at work. After learning about mindful eating, she began practicing slowing down during meals and paying attention to her body's hunger cues. She also started journaling about her stress and seeking healthier ways to manage her emotions, such as taking walks during lunch breaks. Over time, Sarah noticed a significant decrease in emotional eating and started feeling more in control of her relationship with food.

Story 2: Mark's Transformation

Mark had always used food as a reward for both positive and negative emotions. After a stressful day at work, he would turn to fast food as a way to unwind. When he began therapy to address the underlying stress, he realized that food had become a coping mechanism. Mark started implementing stress-reducing activities such as yoga and meditation and gradually reduced his reliance on food for comfort. Today, he feels more balanced and is making healthier choices for both his body and mind.

Overcoming emotional eating is a key part of achieving lasting weight loss. By understanding emotional triggers, learning to differentiate between physical and emotional hunger, and developing practical strategies to cope with stress, boredom, and loneliness, you can begin to break the cycle of emotional eating. Incorporating mindful eating techniques and hearing personal stories of success can provide further motivation as you embark on this journey. Remember, emotional eating is not about food—it's about addressing the emotions that drive your eating behavior and finding healthier ways to respond.

Chapter 4

Building New Habits for Lasting Change

Weight loss isn't just about diet and exercise; it's about developing habits that support a sustainable, healthy lifestyle. Habits shape much of what we do each day, from the food we eat to the way we move. If your habits align with your weight loss goals, success becomes much easier to achieve. However, if your habits work against you, even the best diet or workout plan will fall short in the long term.

This chapter focuses on understanding the science of habit formation, identifying and breaking bad habits related to food and exercise, and offering a step-by-step guide to creating sustainable weight loss habits. We will also explore habit stacking—a powerful tool to anchor new healthy behaviors—and provide practical tips to build daily routines that promote lasting change.

The Science of Habit Formation: How Habits Influence Behavior

Habits are automatic behaviors that we repeat regularly, often without thinking. They are formed through repetition and reinforcement, creating neural pathways in the brain that make certain actions feel natural or instinctive. When it comes to weight loss, your habits—whether healthy or unhealthy—play a crucial role in determining your success.

The process of habit formation is grounded in a psychological model known as the **habit loop,** which consists of three components:

1. **Cue**: A trigger that initiates the behavior.
2. **Routine**: The behavior itself, or the action you take in response to the cue.
3. **Reward**: The positive outcome or satisfaction you receive after completing the behavior, reinforcing the habit.

For example, if you have a habit of snacking while watching TV, the cue might be sitting down in front of the television, the routine is grabbing a snack, and the reward is the satisfaction of eating something tasty while relaxing. Over time, this behavior becomes ingrained, and you may find yourself automatically reaching for snacks every time you turn on the TV, regardless of whether you're physically hungry.

The good news is that habits can be changed. By understanding how habits work, you can start to break bad ones and replace them with healthier alternatives.

Identifying and Breaking Bad Habits Related to Food and Exercise

Before you can build new, healthier habits, it's essential to identify the bad habits that are holding you back. Often, these habits are so ingrained that we don't even realize they're happening. By paying attention to your daily routines and behaviors, you can begin to recognize the habits that are sabotaging your weight loss efforts.

Here are some common bad habits related to food and exercise:

1. **Mindless Eating**: Eating while distracted—whether it's in front of the TV, while scrolling through your phone, or working at your desk—can lead to

overeating. You may consume more food than you need because you're not paying attention to your hunger cues.

2. **Skipping Meals**: Skipping meals, especially breakfast, can slow down your metabolism and lead to overeating later in the day. It can also cause energy crashes, making you more likely to reach for sugary or high-fat snacks for a quick energy boost.

3. **Late-Night Snacking**: Eating late at night, particularly high-calorie snacks, can hinder weight loss by adding extra calories when your body needs less energy. This habit is often driven by boredom, stress, or emotional triggers rather than physical hunger.

4. **Inconsistent Exercise**: Skipping workouts or exercising sporadically can make it difficult to see consistent results. Without regular physical activity, it's

challenging to burn enough calories to support weight loss and maintain a healthy metabolism.

5. **Relying on Processed Foods**: Relying on convenience foods, which are often high in unhealthy fats, sugar, and sodium, can derail your progress. These foods are often low in nutrients, leaving you unsatisfied and more likely to overeat.

How to Break Bad Habits

Breaking a bad habit requires disrupting the habit loop and replacing the old routine with a new, healthier behavior. Here's how to get started:

1. **Identify the Cue**: The first step is to recognize what triggers the habit. Is it a specific time of day, an emotional state, or an environmental factor? For

example, you might notice that you tend to snack when you're feeling bored or anxious.

2. **Analyze the Routine**: Once you've identified the cue, examine the behavior that follows. What action do you take in response to the cue? This could be reaching for a snack, skipping a workout, or eating fast food on your way home from work.

3. **Find a Replacement Behavior**: To break the habit, you need to replace the unhealthy behavior with a healthier alternative. If boredom triggers snacking, try engaging in a different activity, such as taking a walk, reading a book, or calling a friend.

4. **Reinforce the New Habit with a Reward**: Just as the old habit had a reward, you need to create a reward for the new behavior. This could be the

satisfaction of completing a workout, the sense of accomplishment from preparing a healthy meal, or the physical energy boost you feel after making a healthier choice.

By understanding the cues and rewards that drive your bad habits, you can start to rewire your brain and replace them with behaviors that support your weight loss goals.

Step-by-Step Guide to Creating Sustainable Weight Loss Habits

Creating sustainable habits for weight loss requires a strategic approach. It's not just about making temporary changes; it's about establishing new routines that will last a lifetime. Here's a step-by-step guide to help you build sustainable habits for weight loss:

Step 1: Start Small

One of the biggest mistakes people make when trying to form new habits is taking on too much at once. While it's tempting to overhaul your entire lifestyle in one go, this approach is rarely sustainable. Instead, focus on small, manageable changes that are easier to maintain over time. For example:

- Instead of trying to completely cut out junk food, start by reducing your intake gradually.
- Instead of committing to an intense workout regimen right away, start with a 10-minute daily walk and gradually increase the duration and intensity.

Small changes are easier to stick to and help build momentum as you experience early successes.

Step 2: Set Specific, Measurable Goals

Vague goals like "eat healthier" or "exercise more" are difficult to measure and achieve. Instead, set specific, measurable goals that give you clear direction. For example:

- "I will eat one serving of vegetables with lunch and dinner each day."
- "I will walk for 20 minutes every morning, five days a week."

Having clear, specific goals makes it easier to track your progress and stay accountable.

Step 3: Create a Routine

Habits are built through consistency, so it's important to create a routine that you can follow daily. If your goal is to exercise regularly, schedule your workouts at the same time each day, such as first thing in the morning or during your lunch break. If your goal is to eat healthier, plan and prepare your meals at the same time each week.

By establishing a routine, you eliminate the need to make decisions about your habits every day. Instead, your new behaviors become automatic parts of your day.

Step 4: Track Your Progress

Tracking your progress is essential for staying motivated and seeing how far you've come. Use a habit tracker, journal, or app to monitor your daily actions. Whether it's noting how many times you exercised, logging your meals, or tracking your weight loss, keeping a record of your progress helps reinforce the habit and encourages you to keep going.

Step 5: Adjust When Necessary

It's important to recognize that building habits isn't always a linear process. There will be setbacks, and that's okay. If you miss a workout or indulge in an unhealthy meal, don't view it as a failure. Instead, reflect on what led to the setback and adjust your plan if necessary. The key to long-term success is staying flexible and making adjustments when needed.

Using Habit Stacking to Anchor New Healthy Behaviors

One of the most effective strategies for building new habits is **habit stacking**. This technique involves linking a new habit to an existing one, making it easier to incorporate the new behavior into your daily routine.

Here's how habit stacking works:

1. **Identify an Existing Habit**: Choose a habit that you already do consistently,

such as brushing your teeth, making coffee, or commuting to work.

2. **Add a New Habit to the Existing One**: Once you've identified an existing habit, stack a new habit on top of it. For example, if you want to start exercising in the morning, you could stack the new habit onto your existing routine of making coffee. As soon as you finish brewing your coffee, you put on your workout clothes and exercise for 10 minutes.

3. **Repeat Daily**: By consistently pairing the new habit with an established routine, the new behavior becomes automatic over time. The more you repeat the habit stack, the stronger the connection between the two behaviors will become.

Examples of Habit Stacking for Weight Loss

- **Drink Water Before Meals**: Stack the habit of drinking a glass of water with the routine of sitting down to eat. Every time you sit down for a meal, drink a glass of water first.

- **Stretching After Brushing Teeth**: Stack the habit of stretching with brushing your teeth. Every time you brush your teeth, take two minutes to stretch your arms, legs, and back.

- **Meal Prep After Grocery Shopping**: Stack the habit of meal prepping with your grocery shopping routine. As soon as you return from the grocery store, spend 15-20 minutes preparing healthy snacks or portioning out meals for the week.

Habit stacking is a powerful tool because it builds on the momentum of existing routines, making it easier to adopt new behaviors.

Daily Routines for Success: Practical Habit-Building Tips

Success in weight loss is largely a product of your daily routines. Here are practical tips to help you build routines that support your goals:

1. **Plan Your Meals**: Take time each week to plan your meals and snacks. Having a plan in place makes it easier to stick to healthy eating habits and avoid impulsive food choices.

2. **Schedule Your Workouts**: Treat exercise like any other important appointment. Schedule your workouts in advance and commit to them as you would a meeting or deadline.

3. **Set Up Your Environment for Success**: Create an environment that supports your new habits. Keep healthy snacks within reach, clear clutter from your workout space, and remove temptations like sugary snacks from your pantry.

4. **Celebrate Small Wins**: Reward yourself for sticking to your new habits, even if the changes are small. Recognize your progress and celebrate your victories, whether it's by treating yourself to a relaxing activity or simply acknowledging how far you've come.

Building new habits is the foundation of lasting weight loss success. By understanding the science of habit formation, identifying and breaking bad habits, and implementing strategies like habit stacking, you can create routines that support your health goals.

Sustainable change doesn't happen overnight, but with consistency and patience, the new habits you build will become second nature—leading to lasting weight loss and a healthier, happier life.

As James Clear, author of *Atomic Habits*, says: "You do not rise to the level of your goals. You fall to the level of your systems." In the case of weight loss, your systems are your daily habits. Build strong, supportive habits, and success will follow.

Chapter 5

The Motivation Myth: Discipline Over Willpower

When people embark on a weight loss journey, they often rely heavily on willpower, believing that sheer determination will carry them through tough times. However, this approach is flawed. Willpower is a limited resource that can deplete over time, especially when faced with constant temptation or emotional stress. That's why many well-intentioned diets fail— not because people lack the desire to lose weight, but because they rely too much on fleeting willpower and not enough on sustainable discipline and consistency.

This chapter will challenge the common belief that willpower alone can lead to success. Instead, we'll explore how cultivating discipline and building a supportive environment can be more effective. We'll also delve into the importance of setting realistic and meaningful goals that go beyond numbers on the scale, and how to maintain motivation through inevitable setbacks and plateaus.

Why Relying on Willpower Alone Leads to Failure?

Willpower is like a muscle: it gets tired the more you use it. If you're constantly depending on willpower to resist unhealthy food, push through exhaustion for a workout, or avoid temptation, it's only a matter of time before your strength weakens. Psychologists refer to this phenomenon as **ego depletion**, where our capacity for self-control diminishes after repeated use.

Consider the following scenarios:

- You wake up with the best of intentions to eat healthy and exercise. You successfully resist the urge to have a donut for breakfast, say no to the vending machine in the afternoon, and skip dessert at dinner. By evening, you're mentally exhausted from saying "no" all day, and it becomes far easier to give in to a late-night snack craving.

- You start a new diet, highly motivated at first, but as the novelty wears off, the daily struggle of making "good" choices becomes draining. Eventually, you might find yourself binge eating or skipping workouts as your willpower fades.

This is why **willpower** alone isn't a sustainable strategy for weight loss. It's unreliable, inconsistent, and too easily depleted. Success requires something more enduring: **discipline** and **consistent habits** that are built over time.

How to Cultivate Discipline and Consistency?

While willpower might get you through the first few days or weeks of a weight loss program, **discipline** is what keeps you going for the long term. Discipline isn't about perfection or being overly strict with yourself; it's about developing habits and routines that make success almost automatic.

Discipline is like a muscle that strengthens with practice. The more you exercise it, the more reliable and consistent it becomes. Unlike willpower, which fades under stress, discipline creates a solid foundation for lasting change. Here's how you can cultivate it:

1. Create Daily Routines

Routines eliminate the need for constant decision-making and conserve your mental energy. When certain activities—such as preparing meals, exercising, and drinking enough water—become part of your daily routine, you no longer need to rely on motivation to complete them.

- **Actionable step**: Establish a morning routine that includes a healthy breakfast and some form of movement, even if it's just stretching. Plan your meals for the day or week in advance to avoid impulsive choices.

2. Break Big Goals into Smaller Tasks

Discipline is easier to maintain when you're not overwhelmed by massive goals. Break your weight loss journey into smaller, more manageable tasks. For example, instead of focusing on losing 50 pounds, focus on losing 5 pounds at a time. Each small victory fuels your momentum, making it easier to stay disciplined.

- **Actionable step**: Set small weekly goals such as walking an extra 10 minutes each day, cutting out one sugary drink, or adding an extra serving of vegetables to your meals.

3. Embrace the Power of "Non-Negotiables"

Successful people often have "non-negotiables"—habits that they commit to no matter what. Whether it's getting 30 minutes of exercise each day or preparing meals at home, non-negotiables ensure that no matter how tough the day is, your progress continues.

- **Actionable step**: Choose one or two non-negotiables that you commit to daily. For instance, "I will drink at least 8 glasses of water a day," or "I will walk for 20 minutes after dinner."

4. Track Your Progress

Discipline becomes easier when you can see the progress you're making. Tracking your actions reinforces your discipline and gives you tangible evidence of your efforts. This could be as simple as keeping a food journal, logging your workouts, or marking days off on a calendar when you've stuck to your plan.

- **Actionable step**: Use a journal or app to record your meals, workouts, and daily habits. Review it regularly to see how far you've come and where improvements can be made.

Creating a Motivating Environment That Supports Your Weight Loss Goals

Your environment has a profound impact on your behavior. If you're surrounded by temptations, it will be much harder to rely on discipline alone. By creating an environment that supports your goals, you make it easier to stay on track, even when your willpower is low.

Here's how to set yourself up for success:

1. Design Your Kitchen for Healthy Choices

If your kitchen is stocked with unhealthy snacks and junk food, it will take immense discipline to resist them every day. Instead, create a kitchen environment that encourages healthy eating by keeping nutritious foods visible and accessible.

- **Actionable step**: Keep fresh fruits, vegetables, and healthy snacks like nuts or yogurt at eye level in your fridge or pantry. Hide or get rid of high-calorie, low-nutrient foods to minimize temptation.

2. Create a Dedicated Exercise Space

Having a specific area where you exercise—whether it's at home or a gym—makes it easier to stick to your workout routine. This space should be free from distractions and filled with equipment or items that motivate you.

- **Actionable step**: Set up a workout corner at home with a yoga mat, dumbbells, or resistance bands. Play music or listen to a podcast that energizes you during your workouts.

3. Surround Yourself with Support

The people you spend time with can either support or undermine your efforts. Surround yourself with individuals who encourage your progress, hold you accountable, and share your commitment to healthy living.

- **Actionable step**: Join a fitness class, an online community, or find a workout buddy who shares your goals. Engaging with like-minded people can help keep you motivated.

Setting Realistic and Meaningful Goals: Moving Beyond the Scale

One of the most common mistakes people make in their weight loss journey is focusing solely on the number on the scale. While it's natural to want to track your weight, this can often lead to frustration, especially when you hit a plateau or if your progress isn't as fast as expected. Weight fluctuates for many reasons, and it doesn't always reflect the true progress you're making.

Instead, focus on **realistic and meaningful goals** that go beyond the scale. These goals should be specific, achievable, and connected to how you feel, not just how much you weigh.

1. Performance-Based Goals

Rather than focusing on how much weight you've lost, set goals related to physical performance. These goals might include improving your strength, flexibility, or endurance.

- **Actionable step**: Set a goal to be able to do 10 push-ups, run a 5K, or increase the amount of weight you can lift. Celebrate these milestones as signs of progress, regardless of what the scale says.

2. Health-Focused Goals

Weight loss is often about improving overall health, so set goals that reflect positive changes in your well-being. These might include lowering your blood pressure, improving your cholesterol levels, or increasing your energy levels.

- **Actionable step**: Get regular check-ups with your healthcare provider to track health improvements like reduced blood pressure or better cholesterol. Use these results to motivate you, rather than relying solely on weight.

3. Lifestyle Goals

Lifestyle changes are crucial for long-term success, so set goals that reflect positive habits you want to adopt. These might include cooking more meals at home, getting more sleep, or reducing stress.

- **Actionable step**: Set a goal to cook three meals at home per week or to meditate for 10 minutes daily. Track how these lifestyle changes make you feel and contribute to your overall well-being.

How to Stay Motivated During Weight Loss Plateaus and Setbacks

Weight loss plateaus are a normal part of the journey, but they can be incredibly discouraging. After weeks or months of steady progress, it can feel like you've hit a wall when the scale refuses to budge. But plateaus don't mean failure. In fact, they're often a sign that your body is adjusting to its new weight.

Here's how to stay motivated when progress slows or setbacks occur:

1. Focus on Non-Scale Victories

When the scale isn't moving, look for other signs of progress. These might include fitting into smaller clothes, having more energy, sleeping better, or noticing improvements in your mental health.

- **Actionable step**: Keep a journal of non-scale victories. Write down how your clothes fit, how your energy levels have improved, or how much stronger you feel in your workouts.

2. Adjust Your Routine

Sometimes, hitting a plateau means it's time to shake things up. If you've been doing the same workouts or eating the same foods, your body may have adapted. Changing your routine can help you break through the plateau.

- **Actionable step**: Try a new type of exercise, such as strength training, yoga, or interval training. Adjust your eating habits by adding more protein, fiber, or whole foods to your meals.

3. Practice Self-Compassion

Setbacks are inevitable in any weight loss journey. Whether it's overeating, missing workouts, or feeling unmotivated, it's important to be kind to yourself. Progress is not linear, and everyone has ups and downs.

- **Actionable step**: When you experience a setback, avoid harsh self-criticism. Instead, reflect on what led to the setback and how you can learn from it.

Reaffirm your commitment to your
goals and keep moving forward.

The journey to lasting weight loss is not about relying on fleeting bursts of willpower, but about cultivating discipline, building supportive environments, and setting meaningful goals. By focusing on small, achievable steps and embracing the process rather than fixating on the scale, you can create a sustainable path to health and well-being. Plateaus and setbacks are natural parts of the process, but with discipline and the right mindset, they become opportunities for growth, not reasons to give up.

Remember, as author Jim Rohn once said: "Discipline is the bridge between goals and accomplishment." Stay consistent, stay disciplined, and success will follow.

Chapter 6

Visualizing Success: Mental Techniques for Weight Loss

Weight loss is often thought of as a physical process—calories in, calories out. But the truth is, much of the battle happens in the mind. Your thoughts, beliefs, and mental outlook play a pivotal role in whether you succeed or struggle. One of the most powerful mental techniques for success is visualization. Visualization is the practice of imagining yourself achieving your goals, vividly and in detail, to help bring those goals to reality. Combined with affirmations, positive self-talk, and celebrating small victories, these mental techniques can rewire your brain for lasting success.

In this chapter, we'll explore how visualization can be applied to your weight loss journey, offer practical exercises you can incorporate into daily life, and explain how affirmations and positive self-talk can change the way you approach weight loss. Finally, we'll discuss the importance of celebrating small victories as part of your journey to build momentum and stay motivated.

How Visualization Can Help You Achieve Your Weight Loss Goals

Visualization is more than daydreaming—it's an active mental process where you vividly imagine yourself achieving a specific goal. When you practice visualization, you create mental images of what success looks like, feels like, and even tastes like. These images train your brain to recognize what you want and to work towards it, aligning your thoughts, feelings, and actions with your desired outcome.

According to sports psychologists, elite athletes have been using visualization for decades to improve performance. They imagine themselves crossing the finish line, making the perfect shot, or winning the game. This mental rehearsal prepares their brains and bodies for the real event, and it can do the same for you in your weight loss journey.

Here's how visualization helps in weight loss:

1. **Clarifies Your Goals**: When you visualize success, you create a clear and specific image of what you want to achieve. This clarity helps you set more focused, actionable goals. For example, rather than vaguely wanting to "lose

weight," visualization can help you see yourself at a particular weight, wearing a certain size, or engaging in activities you've always wanted to do, like running a marathon or hiking a mountain.

2. **Boosts Motivation**: Visualization taps into the emotional satisfaction of achieving your goal, which can boost motivation. When you picture yourself succeeding, you generate feelings of pride, joy, and confidence. These positive emotions help you stay motivated during challenging moments.

3. **Improves Focus and Consistency**: Visualizing your end goal helps you stay focused on the bigger picture, even when faced with day-to-day temptations or setbacks. It reminds you of why you started and encourages you to stay consistent with your habits.

4. **Rewires Your Brain for Success**:
When you repeatedly visualize yourself succeeding, you create new neural pathways in your brain that reinforce the idea of success. Over time, your brain starts to believe that this version of you is not only possible but inevitable. This is key to overcoming self-doubt and limiting beliefs.

As motivational speaker Tony Robbins says, "Whatever you hold in your mind on a consistent basis is exactly what you will experience in your life." Visualization allows you to hold your goals in your mind, and with practice, it brings those goals to life.

Practical Exercises for Using Visualization in Daily Life

Visualization is a skill that improves with practice. To get the most benefit from it, you should aim to make visualization a daily habit, just like brushing your teeth or preparing your meals. Below are practical exercises for incorporating visualization into your daily routine:

1. Morning Visualization Ritual

Start your day by spending 5–10 minutes visualizing your weight loss success. Find a quiet place where you won't be disturbed, close your eyes, and imagine yourself at your goal weight or fitness level. Picture yourself feeling confident, healthy, and energized. Visualize the changes in your body, your clothing, and your daily activities. Imagine how great it feels to have reached your goal.

- **Practical tip**: Create a clear mental picture by engaging all your senses. What do you see when you look in the mirror? How do your clothes feel on your body? What activities are you able to do that you couldn't do before? The more detailed your visualization, the more powerful it will be.

2. Visualization During Workouts

Visualization can be especially powerful during exercise. As you're working out, imagine yourself becoming stronger, fitter, and closer to your goals with every movement. Visualize the end result you want—whether it's losing a certain amount of weight, running a particular distance, or building muscle.

- **Practical tip**: Use positive self-talk during your workouts, like "I'm getting stronger every day" or "This effort is taking me closer to my goals." Combining visualization with physical effort enhances your mental focus and motivation.

3. *Visualize Overcoming Challenges*

Throughout your weight loss journey, you'll encounter obstacles—temptations, cravings, social situations, or moments of low motivation. One way to prepare for these challenges is to visualize yourself overcoming them before they happen.

- **Practical tip**: If you're going to a social event where unhealthy food will be served, visualize yourself confidently choosing healthier options or politely declining indulgent foods. Picture how proud you'll feel afterward for sticking to your plan. By rehearsing these scenarios mentally, you'll be more likely to succeed in real life.

4. Evening Reflection Visualization

At the end of the day, take a few minutes to reflect on your progress. Visualize how today's actions have brought you closer to your goal. This helps reinforce positive behaviors and motivates you for the next day.

- **Practical tip**: During your evening visualization, celebrate small wins from the day, no matter how minor they seem. Maybe you chose a salad instead of fries, or maybe you walked an extra block on your afternoon walk. Visualize the accumulation of these small wins adding up to big changes over time.

Affirmations and Positive Self-Talk: How They Rewire Your Brain for Success

Affirmations are positive statements that you repeat to yourself, often out loud, to help shift your mindset and overcome limiting beliefs. Combined with positive self-talk, affirmations can rewire your brain for success by replacing negative, self-sabotaging thoughts with empowering ones.

Research shows that the brain is highly malleable. This concept, known as **neuroplasticity**, means that your brain is constantly forming new neural connections based on your thoughts and experiences. By consistently feeding your brain with positive affirmations, you can literally rewire it to support your weight loss journey.

1. The Science Behind Affirmations

Affirmations work by influencing your subconscious mind. Your subconscious doesn't distinguish between reality and imagination—it simply accepts the thoughts and beliefs you feed it. When you repeat positive affirmations regularly, you begin to believe them on a deeper level. This belief shapes your behavior, which ultimately leads to better results.

2. Creating Powerful Affirmations

The key to creating effective affirmations is to focus on statements that are:

- **Positive**: Avoid using words like "don't" or "can't." Focus on what you want to achieve, not what you want to avoid.

- **Present tense**: State your affirmations as if you've already achieved your goal. This reinforces the belief that success is already within your grasp.

- **Specific**: Be clear about what you're affirming. Instead of saying "I am healthy," say "I nourish my body with healthy foods every day."

Examples of weight-loss affirmations include:

- "I am in control of my eating habits."
- "I enjoy exercising and moving my body."
- "I am becoming healthier and more fit every day."
- "I am capable of reaching my weight loss goals."

3. Incorporating Affirmations into Your Daily Routine

To make affirmations effective, you need to repeat them consistently. You can integrate affirmations into your daily routine in several ways:

- **Morning routine**: Start your day by saying your affirmations out loud in front of the mirror. This sets a positive tone for the day and reinforces your commitment to your goals.

- **During exercise**: While working out, repeat affirmations like "I am getting stronger with every step" or "I love how exercise makes me feel."
- **Before meals**: Use affirmations before eating to encourage mindful eating, such as "I choose foods that nourish and energize my body."
- **Evening reflection**: End your day by repeating your affirmations and visualizing your success.

The Importance of Celebrating Small Victories

It's easy to get caught up in the pursuit of big goals, but the truth is, lasting success is built on the accumulation of small victories. Celebrating these wins—no matter how small—helps reinforce positive behaviors, boosts motivation, and keeps you focused on the progress you're making.

1. Why Small Victories Matter

When you celebrate small victories, you activate the brain's reward system, releasing dopamine, a feel-good neurotransmitter that motivates you to keep going. These celebrations create a positive feedback loop: each small win makes you feel good, which makes you want to repeat the behavior that led to that win. Over time, this leads to the development of sustainable habits.

2. How to Recognize Small Victories

Small victories don't have to be monumental achievements. They can be as simple as:

- Choosing a healthy snack over junk food.

- Going for a walk instead of watching TV.
- Drinking enough water for the day.
- Saying "no" to a temptation that would have derailed your progress.
- Completing a workout, even if it wasn't your best.

Each of these actions represents progress, and progress—no matter how small—deserves recognition.

3. Ways to Celebrate Your Wins

Celebrating doesn't mean indulging in unhealthy rewards. Instead, find non-food-related ways to acknowledge your progress, such as:

- **Journaling**: Write down your small wins at the end of each day. Over time, you'll have a record of how far you've come.

- **Reward yourself with self-care**: Treat yourself to something that enhances your well-being, like a massage, a new workout outfit, or a relaxing bath.

- **Share your success**: Tell a friend or family member about your small victory. Sharing your progress with others can increase your sense of accomplishment and reinforce your commitment to your goals.

Visualization, affirmations, and celebrating small victories are powerful mental techniques that can help you achieve lasting success in your weight loss journey. By consistently visualizing your goals, practicing positive self-talk, and recognizing the progress you make each day, you rewire your brain to support your efforts. These techniques may seem simple, but they create profound changes in the way you think, feel, and act.

As you move forward in your journey, remember that the key to success isn't just in the physical actions you take, but in the mental habits you cultivate. Your mind is your greatest asset—use it wisely, and you will achieve the lasting change you desire.

In the words of Dr. Wayne Dyer: "Change the way you look at things, and the things you look at change."

Chapter 7

Overcoming Obstacles and Setbacks

Embarking on a weight loss journey is a commitment that requires both physical and mental strength. While following a healthy eating plan and regular exercise are crucial, the real challenge often lies in dealing with the inevitable obstacles and setbacks that arise. Whether it's a slip-up in your diet, feeling discouraged after a plateau, or succumbing to social pressure, these hurdles can make or break your progress. The difference between those who achieve long-term success and those who give up often boils down to how they handle these setbacks.

In this chapter, we will explore the common mental roadblocks that derail weight loss efforts, practical strategies to bounce back from slip-ups, and the importance of building resilience. Additionally, we'll discuss ways to handle social pressures, temptation, and discouragement, providing you with the mental tools to navigate challenges and turn setbacks into comebacks.

Common Mental Roadblocks to Weight Loss

While physical challenges, like lack of time or access to healthy foods, can impede weight loss, mental roadblocks are often the most insidious obstacles to success. These mental barriers can sabotage your progress if not addressed. Understanding and identifying them is the first step toward overcoming them.

1. Perfectionism

Many people approach weight loss with an all-or-nothing mentality. They believe that if they don't follow their plan perfectly, they've failed. This perfectionist mindset can be detrimental because it leads to discouragement and giving up after even the smallest setback. For example, eating an unhealthy meal might lead to the thought, "I've already blown it, so I might as well give up."

- **Solution**: Shift your mindset to focus on progress, not perfection. Understand that setbacks are a normal part of the process, and one slip-up does not erase your overall progress. Instead of striving for perfection, aim for consistency.

2. Negative Self-Talk

The language you use to talk to yourself has a powerful impact on your success. Many people engage in harsh self-criticism, especially when they don't meet their weight loss goals. Thoughts like "I'll never be able to lose weight," "I'm a failure," or "Why bother trying?" can create a cycle of self-sabotage that undermines your efforts.

- **Solution**: Replace negative self-talk with affirmations and positive language. Instead of saying, "I can't do this," say, "I'm capable of making small changes every day that add up to big results." Rewriting the narrative in your mind can shift your attitude and motivation.

3. Fear of Failure

The fear of not reaching your goals or failing yet another diet can hold you back from even trying. Many people avoid making changes because they are afraid they'll be disappointed. This fear can lead to procrastination, avoidance, and self-sabotage.

- **Solution**: Embrace failure as a learning opportunity. Every setback provides valuable lessons that can inform your future efforts. Instead of fearing failure, view it as part of the process. As motivational speaker Zig Ziglar said, "Failure is an event, not a person."

4. Lack of Patience

Weight loss is a gradual process, but in a world where instant gratification is the norm, it's easy to get frustrated when results don't happen quickly. Impatience can lead to abandoning your efforts when you don't see immediate progress, especially when the scale doesn't move as fast as you'd like.

- **Solution**: Focus on the long game. Weight loss is not a race, and sustainable results take time. Celebrate small wins and non-scale victories, like increased energy, improved fitness, or healthier habits. These markers of progress are just as important as the number on the scale.

How to Bounce Back from Slip-Ups and Failures

No matter how disciplined you are, slip-ups are inevitable. Whether you overindulge at a social event, skip a workout, or experience a prolonged plateau, how you respond to these setbacks is what matters most. Bouncing back from failures is a skill that can be learned and strengthened with practice.

1. Acknowledge the Setback Without Guilt

When you experience a setback, it's important to acknowledge it without attaching guilt or shame to it. Feeling guilty about slipping up only serves to reinforce negative emotions and can lead to further poor choices. Instead, acknowledge the setback as a natural part of the journey.

- **Practical step**: After a slip-up, take a few moments to reflect on what happened. Ask yourself, "What led to this setback? How can I avoid this situation in the future?" This reflection helps you learn from the experience without dwelling on guilt.

2. Get Back on Track Quickly

One of the most common mistakes people make after a setback is allowing it to derail their entire plan. A single unhealthy meal can turn into a weekend of overindulgence, which can spiral into giving up altogether. The key is to get back on track as soon as possible.

- **Practical step**: Don't wait for Monday to start again. The moment you recognize the setback, take action to correct course. If you overate at lunch, make a healthy choice for dinner. If you missed a workout, commit to moving your body the next day. The quicker you bounce back, the less impact the setback will have on your progress.

3. Practice Self-Compassion

Treat yourself with the same kindness and understanding that you would offer a friend in a similar situation. Research shows that people who practice self-compassion are more likely to stay motivated and resilient in the face of challenges. Beating yourself up over a setback only increases stress and makes it harder to stay on track.

- **Practical step**: When you slip up, remind yourself that no one is perfect and that setbacks are part of the process. Use affirmations like "I am learning from this experience" or "This is a temporary setback, not a permanent failure."

4. Refocus on Your Why

When setbacks happen, it's easy to lose sight of why you started your weight loss journey in the first place. Reconnecting with your "why" can reignite your motivation and help you move past the setback.

- **Practical step**: Write down the reasons you want to lose weight and keep them somewhere visible. Whether it's improving your health, boosting your confidence, or setting an example for your family, these reasons will remind you of the bigger picture when challenges arise.

Developing Resilience: Turning Setbacks into Comebacks

Resilience is the ability to bounce back from adversity, and it's a critical skill for anyone on a weight loss journey. Developing resilience involves cultivating a mindset that views challenges as opportunities for growth, rather than reasons to give up.

1. Shift Your Mindset

Instead of seeing setbacks as failures, view them as part of the learning process. Every challenge you encounter offers a chance to learn something new about yourself and your habits. This shift in mindset helps you build resilience and stay committed, even when things don't go according to plan.

- **Practical step**: When faced with a setback, ask yourself, "What can I learn from this experience?" By focusing on the lessons, rather than the disappointment, you'll be better equipped to avoid the same pitfalls in the future.

2. Setbacks Are Temporary

One of the most important aspects of resilience is understanding that setbacks are temporary. A bad week doesn't define your entire journey. By keeping setbacks in perspective, you can maintain a sense of control and continue moving forward.

- **Practical step**: When you experience a setback, remind yourself that it's just a small bump in the road. Use phrases like "This too shall pass" to remind yourself that setbacks are temporary and don't define your overall progress.

3. Celebrate Your Resilience

Overcoming obstacles and bouncing back from setbacks are accomplishments in themselves. Every time you get back on track after a slip-up, you're building resilience and strengthening your ability to succeed in the long run.

- **Practical step**: When you recover from a setback, take a moment to celebrate your resilience. Acknowledge the effort it took to get back on track, and recognize that this is a victory worth celebrating.

Practical Strategies for Dealing with Social Pressures, Temptation, and Discouragement

External factors, like social pressures and temptation, can be just as challenging as internal roadblocks. Learning how to navigate these situations with confidence and grace is essential for long-term success.

1. Dealing with Social Pressures

Social events, family gatherings, and holidays often revolve around food, and it can be difficult to stick to your weight loss plan in these situations. Well-meaning friends or family members might encourage you to indulge, making it harder to stay on track.

- **Practical step**: Plan ahead before social events. If possible, bring a healthy dish to share, or review the menu in advance if you're dining out. Practice polite but firm responses for when people offer food that doesn't align with your goals, such as, "Thank you, but I'm focusing on making healthier choices right now."

2. Managing Temptation

Temptation is a part of life, whether it's in the form of a sweet treat at the office or a late-night craving for comfort food. The key is not to avoid temptation entirely, but to manage it in a way that supports your goals.

- **Practical step**: When you feel tempted, pause and ask yourself, "Is this going to bring me closer to my goal?" This moment of reflection can help you make more mindful choices. If you do choose to indulge, enjoy the treat mindfully without guilt, and then get back on track with your next meal.

3. Staying Motivated During Discouragement

Weight loss plateaus, slow progress, or external criticism can lead to discouragement, making it hard to stay motivated. During these times, it's important to remember that the journey is about more than just the number on the scale.

- **Practical step**: Keep a journal of non-scale victories, like increased energy, better sleep, or improved mood. Reflecting on these positive changes can help you stay motivated when progress feels slow. Additionally, surround yourself with a supportive community that uplifts and encourages you.

Overcoming obstacles and setbacks is a vital part of the weight loss journey. Whether you're dealing with internal roadblocks like perfectionism and negative self-talk, or external challenges like social pressures and temptation, learning to navigate these hurdles is key to long-term success. By bouncing back from slip-ups, developing resilience, and employing practical strategies to handle difficult situations, you'll be able to stay on track and turn setbacks into comebacks. As you continue your journey, remember that every challenge is an opportunity for growth, and with the right mindset, you can overcome any obstacle in your path.

In the words of Nelson Mandela: "Do not judge me by my successes, judge me by how many times I fell down and got back up again."

Chapter 8

Creating a Support System

Losing weight is often seen as a solitary journey, one where discipline, diet, and exercise take center stage. However, social support is a crucial, yet frequently overlooked, aspect of long-term weight loss success. A strong support system can provide motivation, accountability, encouragement, and advice during challenging times. In fact, research consistently shows that people who have a positive network of friends, family, or even professional help tend to stick to their weight loss goals longer and achieve better results.

This chapter delves into the importance of social support in weight loss, how to build a positive network, finding communities for encouragement and accountability, and when it's necessary to seek professional help through coaching or therapy. By the end of this chapter, you'll be equipped with actionable steps to create your own personalized support system that will serve as a foundation for lasting change.

The Role of Social Support in Weight Loss Success

Weight loss isn't just a physical challenge—it's an emotional and psychological one too. As with any major lifestyle change, having a network of supportive people can make all the difference. Whether it's family, friends, or a professional coach, the people around you can significantly influence your behavior, mindset, and outcomes.

1. Accountability: A Key to Consistency

One of the greatest benefits of having a support system is accountability. When you know others are invested in your journey, it becomes harder to backslide or give up. Accountability partners or groups can help you stay on track by regularly checking in on your progress, offering motivation, and reminding you of your goals. Knowing that someone is rooting for your success encourages you to keep pushing, even when your motivation wanes.

- **Actionable step**: Find someone you trust to be your accountability partner. Schedule regular check-ins where you can discuss your progress, challenges, and successes. This could be a friend, family member, or even someone online who shares similar goals.

2. Emotional Support in Tough Times

Weight loss is not always a linear journey. There will be ups and downs, and during those low moments, having someone to provide emotional support can prevent you from giving up. A kind word, a shared experience, or even a listening ear can help alleviate feelings of discouragement or frustration. Emotional support can also come in the form of celebrating your victories, no matter how small, and reminding you of how far you've come.

- **Actionable step**: Communicate your needs to those in your support system. Let them know when you're struggling or when you need encouragement. Don't be afraid to ask for help, whether it's a pep talk or someone to join you on a walk.

3. Practical Guidance and Advice

Sometimes, those in your support network can provide practical advice based on their own experiences. Whether it's sharing recipes, workout routines, or time management tips, having someone who has walked the same path can provide valuable insights. Learning from the successes and mistakes of others can accelerate your own progress.

- **Actionable step**: Seek out people who have successfully lost weight and maintained it. Ask them about their strategies and approaches. Their guidance can offer new perspectives and tips that you may not have considered.

4. Creating a Sense of Belonging

Feeling connected to others who are on a similar journey can create a sense of belonging that enhances motivation. Whether it's an online group or a local fitness class, being part of a community of like-minded individuals reminds you that you're not alone. This sense of camaraderie fosters a more positive experience, as you're surrounded by people who understand your struggles and cheer on your victories.

- **Actionable step**: Join a community focused on weight loss or healthy living. This can be a fitness class, an online forum, or a support group. Being part of a collective effort can provide an extra layer of motivation.

How to Build a Positive Network of Friends, Family, and Accountability Partners?

A strong support system doesn't happen by accident—it requires deliberate effort to build. While some people are fortunate to have supportive friends and family already in place, others may need to seek out new relationships or foster deeper connections with those around them. Here's how to build a network that helps you stay focused on your goals.

1. Identify Supportive Individuals

The first step to building a positive network is identifying the people who are genuinely supportive of your goals. These are the individuals who encourage you, provide constructive feedback, and respect the changes you're making in your life. It's also important to recognize that not everyone will understand or support your weight loss journey, and that's okay. Focus on those who uplift and motivate you.

- **Actionable step**: Make a list of people who you feel could be a part of your support system. Reach out to them individually and share your goals. Let them know how they can best support you, whether through accountability, encouragement, or just being a sounding board.

2. Communicate Your Needs Clearly

One of the most common mistakes people make when seeking support is assuming others know what they need. Your friends and family may want to help, but they may not understand how to do so effectively. Clear communication is essential for getting the support you need.

- **Actionable step**: Be specific when discussing your goals and challenges. For example, if you need someone to join you on a daily walk, ask directly. If you'd prefer not to be offered certain foods at family gatherings, kindly express that. Clarity reduces misunderstandings and ensures that your support system is truly helpful.

3. Set Boundaries with Unsupportive Individuals

Unfortunately, not everyone in your life will be supportive of your weight loss efforts. Some may unintentionally undermine your progress by encouraging unhealthy habits or making negative comments. In these situations, setting boundaries is crucial for protecting your progress.

- **Actionable step**: Politely but firmly communicate your boundaries. For instance, if someone frequently encourages you to eat unhealthy food, you might say, "I'm really focusing on my health right now, and I'd appreciate it if we could avoid those types of conversations." Boundaries help protect your mental space and keep you focused on your goals.

4. Strengthen Accountability

Accountability is one of the most effective tools in your support system. Whether it's checking in with a friend, joining a weight loss challenge, or participating in a workout group, consistent accountability helps keep you on track.

- **Actionable step**: Schedule regular accountability check-ins. These could be weekly or bi-weekly meetings with a friend or accountability partner where you discuss your progress, set new goals, and review challenges. This structure creates a sense of responsibility that motivates you to stay consistent.

Finding Like-Minded Communities: Online and Offline Resources for Support

In today's digital world, it's easier than ever to find communities that align with your weight loss goals. Whether you prefer in-person connections or virtual groups, being part of a like-minded community can provide additional layers of support, motivation, and inspiration.

1. Online Communities and Forums

The internet is filled with weight loss communities that cater to various interests and approaches. Whether you're following a specific diet or just looking for general health advice, online forums and social media groups allow you to connect with others who share your goals. These platforms offer a space to ask questions, share progress, and find encouragement from people around the world.

- **Actionable step**: Join a few online weight loss communities that resonate with you. Look for active, positive groups where members are supportive and non-judgmental. Facebook groups, Reddit forums, and dedicated health platforms like My FitnessPal have thriving communities for those seeking support.

2. In-Person Support Groups

In-person support groups can offer a deeper sense of connection and accountability than online groups. Being able to meet face-to-face with others on a similar journey creates a sense of community that can be incredibly motivating. Weight loss groups like Weight Watchers (WW) or local fitness classes are examples of in-person support systems that encourage accountability and shared experiences.

- **Actionable step**: Research local weight loss groups or fitness classes in your area. Many community centers, gyms, and health clubs offer weight loss support groups or meetups where you can connect with others in person. The sense of camaraderie from in-person interactions can help boost motivation.

3. Using Technology for Support

Technology can also be a powerful tool in your support system. Apps that track your progress, send reminders, or connect you with others who share similar goals can provide an extra layer of motivation. From step-counting apps to nutrition trackers, technology makes it easier than ever to stay on track.

- **Actionable step**: Download a health-tracking app that offers community features or challenges. Apps like Fitbit, Noom, and My FitnessPal allow you to connect with friends, join challenges, and track your progress in real time.

Coaching and Therapy: When and How to Seek Professional Help

Sometimes, building a support system requires seeking professional help in the form of coaching or therapy. Coaches and therapists can provide the structured guidance, accountability, and emotional support needed to overcome deeper challenges or mental roadblocks.

1. The Role of a Weight Loss Coach

A weight loss coach is trained to help you set realistic goals, develop personalized strategies, and stay accountable. Coaches often offer one-on-one sessions where they provide advice tailored to your specific needs, whether it's nutrition, exercise, or mental motivation. Having a coach can be particularly helpful if you've struggled to stay consistent or need more structure in your approach.

- **Actionable step**: If you feel like you've hit a plateau or need additional guidance, consider hiring a weight loss coach. Many coaches offer virtual sessions, making it convenient to find one that suits your needs. When selecting a coach, look for someone with a proven track record and a style that resonates with you.

2. Therapy for Emotional and Psychological Support

Weight loss is not just about diet and exercise—it's often deeply connected to emotional and psychological issues. For those dealing with emotional eating, low self-esteem, or past trauma, therapy can be a transformative tool. A therapist can help you identify underlying issues, address mental roadblocks, and develop healthier coping mechanisms.

- **Actionable step**: If emotional or psychological issues are affecting your weight loss journey, seek the help of a licensed therapist who specializes in health or eating behaviors. Therapy can help you address the root causes of emotional eating, self-sabotage, or other mental barriers that hinder your progress.

3. Group Coaching and Counseling

If one-on-one coaching or therapy isn't for you, consider group coaching or counseling. Group settings provide a sense of community while still offering the guidance of a professional. Many weight loss groups offer group coaching sessions where participants can share experiences, challenges, and strategies under the guidance of a trained coach or counselor.

- **Actionable step**: Look for group coaching programs or counseling sessions in your area or online. Many wellness centers and therapy practices offer group programs designed for weight loss or healthy living.

Building a support system is one of the most powerful things you can do to ensure long-term weight loss success. Whether it's leaning on friends and family, joining a community of like-minded individuals, or seeking professional help, having a network of support can provide the accountability, encouragement, and guidance needed to stay on track. Remember, weight loss is not just a solo journey—it's one that's made easier when you have people by your side who want to see you succeed.

In the words of Helen Keller, "Alone we can do so little; together we can do so much."

Chapter 9

Developing a Sustainable Relationship with Food

When embarking on a weight loss journey, many people develop a complicated relationship with food—one often marked by guilt, anxiety, or rigid restrictions. This mindset can lead to unhealthy patterns, such as yo-yo dieting, emotional eating, or an "all-or-nothing" mentality. Developing a sustainable relationship with food is essential for long-term success, allowing you to enjoy eating without fear, and maintain your progress in a balanced, mindful way.

This chapter will explore the ways to cultivate a healthier relationship with food by discussing how to enjoy food without guilt, the importance of creating balance through strategies like the 80/20 rule, the practice of intuitive eating, and practical tips for meal planning and portion control. Additionally, we'll dive into personal success stories from individuals who have found food freedom through these techniques.

How to Enjoy Food Without Guilt or Anxiety?

One of the biggest mental roadblocks in developing a healthy relationship with food is the guilt or anxiety that often accompanies eating, especially when consuming so-called "unhealthy" foods. Many people associate food with judgment—labeling some foods as "good" and others as "bad." This binary thinking can lead to guilt when eating anything deemed "bad," which, in turn, can cause stress and negative emotions.

1. Reframing Your Relationship with Food

The first step to enjoying food without guilt is shifting your mindset from restriction and punishment to one of nourishment and balance. Food is not the enemy, but a source of energy, pleasure, and sustenance. Instead of labeling foods as good or bad, view them on a spectrum, understanding that some foods offer more nutrients and benefits, while others can still be enjoyed in moderation.

- **Actionable Step**: Practice mindful language around food. Instead of saying "I can't eat that," try "I choose to eat this because it nourishes me" or "I'm enjoying this treat because I deserve balance in my life." Changing the language you use helps reduce anxiety and creates a healthier mindset.

2. Allowing Room for Treats

It's important to understand that indulging in your favorite foods doesn't mean you've failed. In fact, allowing yourself to enjoy occasional treats can prevent the binge-restrict cycle that often occurs when we try to eliminate certain foods completely. A sustainable relationship with food involves understanding that indulgences are part of life and don't negate your overall progress.

- **Actionable Step**: Designate moments for treats without guilt. Whether it's a small piece of chocolate after dinner or a weekend brunch with friends, allow yourself to enjoy the experience without obsessing over the calories or feeling like you've "ruined" your diet.

Creating a Balanced Approach to Eating: The 80/20 Rule

One of the most effective strategies for developing a sustainable relationship with food is the 80/20 rule. This approach encourages you to eat nutritious, whole foods 80% of the time while allowing for flexibility and indulgence the remaining 20%. The 80/20 rule removes the pressure of perfection and fosters a balanced, enjoyable approach to eating.

1. Why the 80/20 Rule Works

The reason many diets fail is that they are too restrictive, making it difficult to stick with them long-term. The 80/20 rule eliminates the need for such rigidity. By focusing on making healthy choices most of the time, you're still able to enjoy less nutritious foods in moderation without feeling like you've fallen off track.

- **Actionable Step**: Begin by assessing your current eating habits. Aim to fill your meals with whole, nutrient-dense foods like fruits, vegetables, lean proteins, and whole grains 80% of the time. The other 20% can include less nutritious options like pizza, dessert, or other indulgences. This flexibility allows for a more balanced lifestyle and reduces feelings of deprivation.

2. Practical Application of the 80/20 Rule

Implementing the 80/20 rule can be as simple as ensuring that most of your meals are nutrient-rich while allowing yourself small indulgences throughout the week. This could mean choosing healthier options during the workweek and indulging a little more on the weekends.

- **Actionable Step**: Plan your week with the 80/20 rule in mind. For instance, eat balanced meals Monday through Friday, focusing on whole foods. Then, on Saturday night, treat yourself to a favorite dish or dessert. This approach helps you stay consistent without feeling deprived.

Intuitive Eating: Listening to Your Body's Cues

Intuitive eating is a practice that encourages you to listen to your body's natural hunger and fullness cues rather than following external dieting rules. This approach rejects the diet mentality and teaches you to trust your body, eat when you're hungry, and stop when you're satisfied. Intuitive eating is not about following a meal plan or calorie counting, but rather about tuning into your body's needs.

1. The Principles of Intuitive Eating

At its core, intuitive eating is about making peace with food and learning to respond to your body's signals of hunger and fullness. It involves rejecting the idea that food should be restricted and instead focusing on internal cues to guide your eating behavior.

- **Actionable Step**: The next time you sit down for a meal, check in with yourself. Are you truly hungry, or are you eating out of boredom or stress? Practice pausing halfway through your meal to assess how full you feel. If you're satisfied, stop eating. If you're still hungry, continue. This practice helps develop body awareness.

2. Rejecting the Diet Mentality

Many people struggle with intuitive eating because they've been conditioned by years of dieting to ignore their hunger cues. Diet culture often promotes the idea that certain foods should be avoided or that hunger should be ignored. Intuitive eating encourages you to trust that your body knows what it needs.

- **Actionable Step**: Begin by rejecting any lingering diet rules in your life. Stop labeling foods as off-limits or feeling like you must adhere to strict eating times. Instead, focus on how your body feels and respond accordingly. Trust that your body is capable of guiding you toward the right balance of food.

3. Overcoming Emotional Eating

One of the challenges in practicing intuitive eating is distinguishing between physical hunger and emotional hunger. Emotional hunger is when we eat in response to feelings like stress, boredom, sadness, or even happiness, rather than because our body needs nourishment. Learning to differentiate between these types of hunger is key to successful intuitive eating.

- **Actionable Step**: The next time you find yourself reaching for food, ask yourself: "Am I physically hungry or emotionally hungry?" If it's the latter, explore non-food ways to manage your emotions, such as taking a walk, journaling, or talking to a friend.

Practical Tips for Meal Planning and Portion Control

Developing a sustainable relationship with food doesn't mean ignoring structure altogether. Meal planning and portion control are essential tools that can help you maintain balance and avoid overeating, especially when life gets busy. These practices create a foundation for consistency and ensure that you're nourishing your body in a way that aligns with your goals.

1. The Benefits of Meal Planning

Meal planning helps reduce the temptation to make impulsive, less healthy food choices. When you take the time to plan your meals ahead of time, you have greater control over the ingredients and portion sizes, and you're less likely to reach for convenience foods that don't align with your goals.

- **Actionable Step**: Set aside time each week to plan your meals. This doesn't mean you have to prepare every meal in advance, but having a plan ensures that you have healthy options available. Consider batch cooking or prepping ingredients for easy assembly throughout the week.

2. Portion Control Without Feeling Deprived

Portion control is not about restricting yourself—it's about eating the right amount of food for your body's needs. Many people unintentionally overeat because they're unaware of portion sizes or eat directly from large containers. Learning to serve appropriate portions can help you avoid overeating while still feeling satisfied.

- **Actionable Step**: Use smaller plates and bowls to help control portion sizes without feeling deprived. Visual cues like filling half your plate with vegetables can help guide portion sizes naturally. Another strategy is to serve meals in the kitchen rather than placing all the food on the table, which reduces the temptation for second helpings.

3. Mindful Eating Practices

Meal planning and portion control work best when combined with mindful eating. This involves slowing down, savoring each bite, and paying attention to your body's signals. Mindful eating helps prevent overeating and allows you to enjoy your food more fully.

- **Actionable Step**: During your next meal, remove distractions like your phone or television. Focus on the colors, textures, and flavors of your food. Chew slowly, and take note of how you feel as you eat. This practice can help you recognize when you're satisfied and prevent overeating.

Personal Anecdotes: Readers' Success Stories on Finding Food Freedom

Many people have successfully transformed their relationship with food, moving from a place of restriction and guilt to one of balance and freedom. These personal stories illustrate that finding food freedom is not only possible but sustainable.

1. Samantha's Journey to Intuitive Eating

Samantha struggled with yo-yo dieting for years. Every time she started a new diet, she would lose a few pounds, but eventually, the restrictions would lead to binge eating. After discovering intuitive eating, Samantha learned to listen to her body's hunger cues and honor her cravings without guilt. Over time, she stopped bingeing and found a weight that felt healthy and sustainable.

Her advice to others is to "Trust the process. It took me time to learn how to listen to my body, but once I did, I realized I didn't need to diet anymore. I can enjoy food without guilt, and that's true freedom."

2. John's Success with the 80/20 Rule

John was always an all-or-nothing eater. He'd go on strict diets where he'd eliminate all his favorite foods, only to binge on them after a few weeks. After learning about the 80/20 rule, John began incorporating balance into his eating. He focused on healthy meals during the week and allowed himself to enjoy indulgences on the weekends.

"The 80/20 rule was a game changer for me," John says. "I realized I didn't have to be perfect all the time to maintain a healthy lifestyle. Now I can enjoy pizza with friends without feeling like I've failed.

Developing a sustainable relationship with food is about balance, mindfulness, and trust. It's about enjoying food without guilt, understanding your body's needs, and creating healthy habits that last a lifetime. Whether through the 80/20 rule, intuitive eating, or meal planning, the goal is to build a foundation that allows you to nourish your body and enjoy your life.

As you continue on your journey, remember the words of Michael Pollan: "Eat food. Not too much. Mostly plants." Let this simple mantra guide your choices and help you cultivate a lasting, positive relationship with food.

Chapter 10

The Mind-Body Connection: Movement and Mental Health

Movement and physical activity have long been associated with physical health benefits like weight loss, improved cardiovascular function, and stronger muscles. However, the connection between movement and mental health is equally powerful and essential. Regular exercise does more than just tone the body—it sharpens the mind, boosts mood, and enhances emotional balance.

This chapter explores how regular exercise can improve mental clarity and emotional well-being, the importance of finding joy in movement, and practical strategies for staying consistent with your exercise routine. Additionally, we'll discuss how to use exercise as a powerful tool for managing stress and boosting mood.

How Regular Exercise Affects Mental Clarity, Focus, and Emotional Balance

The mind and body are intrinsically connected, and physical activity has profound effects on brain function and emotional well-being. Exercise impacts cognitive performance, emotional stability, and overall mental health in several ways.

1. Boosting Mental Clarity and Focus

Engaging in regular physical activity increases blood flow to the brain, which enhances cognitive function and helps you think more clearly. Research has shown that exercise can improve memory, concentration, and attention. The release of chemicals like brain-derived neurotrophic factor (BDNF) during exercise also supports brain health by promoting the growth of new neurons, which strengthens neural connections.

- **Practical Tip**: Incorporate short, brisk walks or stretches into your workday. Even 10-15 minutes of movement can help clear mental fog and refocus your attention on the task at hand. Use exercise as a mental reset throughout your day.

2. Regulating Mood and Emotions

Exercise has a profound effect on emotional regulation due to its impact on neurotransmitters like serotonin, dopamine, and endorphins. These chemicals play a crucial role in enhancing mood and reducing symptoms of anxiety and depression. Physical activity acts as a natural mood stabilizer, helping you manage stress and prevent emotional highs and lows.

- **Practical Tip**: When feeling stressed or overwhelmed, engage in moderate-intensity exercise, such as jogging or cycling. This can lead to an immediate mood boost and help you regain emotional balance.

3. Reducing Stress and Anxiety

Exercise helps reduce levels of cortisol, the body's stress hormone, and encourages relaxation. Regular movement has also been linked to improved sleep, which further supports stress reduction and emotional health. Over time, maintaining an active lifestyle can make you more resilient to the daily stressors of life, improving your capacity to handle difficult situations calmly.

- **Practical Tip**: Develop a habit of exercising when you start to feel anxious or stressed. Whether it's yoga, walking, or strength training, movement can be a powerful way to mitigate anxiety and restore a sense of calm.

Finding Joy in Movement: Choosing Activities That Suit Your Personality and Lifestyle

One of the biggest challenges in establishing a regular exercise routine is finding activities that you genuinely enjoy. When exercise feels like a chore or punishment, it's much harder to stay consistent. On the other hand, when you find joy in movement, it becomes something you look forward to rather than dread.

1. Understanding Your Preferences

To find the right form of exercise, it's important to consider your personality, lifestyle, and preferences. Do you enjoy structured workouts or more spontaneous activities? Do you prefer socializing while exercising or working out alone? Matching your exercise choices to your personality can make the experience more enjoyable and sustainable.

- **Practical Tip**: Try different forms of movement until you find something that resonates with you. This could include dancing, swimming, hiking, or group fitness classes. Listen to your body and your instincts—if a certain activity brings you joy, prioritize it in your routine.

2. Incorporating Fun into Fitness

Fun and enjoyment should be key components of your exercise routine. If you dread going to the gym, it's unlikely you'll maintain that habit long-term. Instead, look for activities that align with your interests and make movement enjoyable. Play a sport, join a dance class, or explore outdoor activities like hiking or cycling. The more enjoyable the activity, the more likely you'll stick with it.

- **Practical Tip**: Create an exercise playlist with your favorite upbeat songs, or invite a friend to join you in an activity you both enjoy. Adding a social element or listening to music can make your workout feel less like a task and more like an enjoyable experience.

3. Adapting Exercise to Your Lifestyle

Exercise doesn't have to fit into the traditional one-hour gym session format. Movement can be integrated into your daily routine in small, manageable ways. The key is to choose activities that complement your lifestyle and schedule, ensuring you make movement a natural part of your day.

- **Practical Tip**: Incorporate movement into your day by taking the stairs instead of the elevator, walking during phone calls, or doing bodyweight exercises during TV commercials. These small bouts of movement can add up to significant health benefits over time.

Practical Strategies for Staying Consistent with Exercise Routines

Consistency is one of the most critical factors for achieving the mental and physical benefits of exercise. However, life's demands can make it difficult to maintain a regular workout routine. By implementing practical strategies, you can stay on track and build lasting exercise habits.

1. Set Realistic and Specific Goals

One reason people fall off their exercise routine is that they set unrealistic goals, such as working out every day or losing a specific amount of weight in a short time. To stay consistent, focus on setting achievable goals that align with your lifestyle. Small, attainable goals build momentum and encourage long-term success.

- **Practical Tip**: Instead of aiming to exercise every day, start with a more realistic goal, like working out three times a week for 30 minutes. Once you've successfully maintained that, you can gradually increase the frequency or duration of your workouts.

2. Make Exercise a Non-Negotiable Part of Your Schedule

One way to ensure you stay consistent with exercise is by treating it like any other important appointment in your schedule. Rather than waiting until you "feel like it," commit to a specific time for your workouts and stick to it.

- **Practical Tip**: Block out time for exercise on your calendar, just like you would for a work meeting or doctor's appointment. Consistently showing up for yourself helps solidify the habit and creates a sense of accountability.

3. Use Habit Stacking to Anchor Your Routine

Habit stacking is a method where you link a new habit (exercise) to an existing habit. For instance, if you always have your morning coffee at the same time, you can stack your exercise routine immediately afterward. This technique makes it easier to incorporate new habits into your day because they're connected to something you already do.

- **Practical Tip**: Identify an existing habit in your daily routine, such as brushing your teeth or making your morning coffee. After completing that task, immediately follow it up with your exercise routine, whether it's a quick 10-minute yoga session or a 30-minute walk.

Using Exercise as a Tool for Managing Stress and Boosting Mood

Exercise is one of the most effective tools for managing stress and improving your mood. It not only reduces cortisol levels, but also stimulates the production of endorphins—your brain's "feel-good" chemicals. Movement allows you to release pent-up energy, clear your mind, and enhance emotional well-being.

1. Exercise as a Stress Reliever

Physical activity serves as a powerful outlet for stress, allowing your body to release tension. Whether through cardiovascular exercise, strength training, or stretching, movement provides both physical and emotional release. Over time, regular exercise can help you build resilience against stress, making it easier to cope with life's challenges.

- **Practical Tip**: When you're feeling overwhelmed, go for a brisk walk or try a 10-minute yoga session. Even short bouts of movement can help shift your mental state, providing immediate relief from stress.

2. Boosting Mood with Regular Movement

One of the most well-known benefits of exercise is its ability to elevate mood. Exercise stimulates the production of endorphins, which can lead to a feeling of euphoria commonly referred to as the "runner's high." Regular exercise also increases serotonin and dopamine levels, which help improve mood, reduce anxiety, and ward off depression.

- **Practical Tip**: Include a form of movement that makes you happy in your daily routine. Whether it's dancing, cycling, or taking a nature walk, choose activities that make you feel good. This can turn exercise into something you look forward to rather than a chore.

3. Mind-Body Exercises for Mental Health

In addition to traditional forms of exercise like running or strength training, mind-body practices such as yoga, tai chi, and pilates offer unique benefits for mental health. These forms of movement focus on breath control, mindfulness, and gentle stretching, all of which can reduce stress and anxiety while enhancing relaxation.

- **Practical Tip**: Incorporate mind-body exercises like yoga or meditation into your routine to support emotional balance. Even just 10 minutes of mindful movement can reduce stress and help you feel more centered throughout the day.

The mind-body connection is a powerful tool for achieving mental clarity, emotional balance, and overall well-being. Regular exercise enhances brain function, improves mood, and reduces stress, making it an essential component of a healthy lifestyle. By finding joy in movement, staying consistent with your routine, and using exercise to manage stress, you can build a sustainable practice that benefits both your body and your mind.

Remember, the key to lasting success is finding activities that you enjoy and can sustain. As you continue your journey, embrace the fact that movement isn't just about losing weight—it's about nourishing your mind and body, creating balance, and fostering resilience. Through consistency and intention, you can harness the power of exercise to elevate your life and mental well-being.

Chapter 11

Mindfulness and Meditation for Weight Loss

In the journey toward achieving lasting weight loss, many people focus on diet and exercise but often overlook the psychological and emotional aspects of their relationship with food. Mindfulness and meditation provide powerful tools for addressing the mental and emotional factors that contribute to overeating, stress, and unhealthy habits. These practices allow individuals to become more in tune with their bodies, recognize their true hunger signals, and manage emotional triggers that lead to overeating.

This chapter will explore how mindfulness practices support weight loss, introduce simple mindfulness and meditation exercises to curb cravings and manage stress, and demonstrate the benefits of deep breathing, yoga, and relaxation techniques in maintaining focus and discipline. We'll also highlight real-life examples of people who have successfully used mindfulness to achieve their weight loss goals.

How Mindfulness Practices Support Weight Loss

Mindfulness, at its core, is the practice of being present and fully engaged in the current moment without judgment. When applied to weight loss, mindfulness helps individuals become more aware of their eating habits, emotional triggers, and physical sensations of hunger and fullness. This awareness is key to breaking the cycle of mindless eating and emotional overeating.

1. Increasing Awareness of Eating Habits

Many people eat on autopilot—mindlessly snacking while watching TV or consuming large portions without realizing it. Mindfulness brings attention to what, why, and how much you're eating. It encourages you to slow down and savor each bite, allowing your body time to signal fullness and satisfaction. By becoming more mindful of your eating habits, you can make more intentional choices that support your weight loss goals.

- **Practical Tip**: Before starting a meal, take a moment to assess your hunger on a scale of 1 to 10. Are you truly hungry, or are you eating out of habit or emotion? By pausing to reflect on your hunger levels, you can make more mindful decisions about when and what to eat.

2. Managing Emotional Eating

Mindfulness also helps individuals recognize the difference between physical hunger and emotional hunger. Emotional hunger is often triggered by stress, boredom, loneliness, or other feelings, leading to overeating as a coping mechanism. By practicing mindfulness, you can identify the emotions driving your desire to eat and respond to them in healthier ways, such as through meditation, deep breathing, or other self-care practices.

- **Practical Tip**: When you feel the urge to eat but aren't physically hungry, pause and ask yourself: "What am I feeling right now? Am I using food to soothe an emotional need?" Acknowledging your emotions can help you address them without turning to food.

3. *Building a Positive Relationship with Food*

Mindfulness encourages a non-judgmental approach to eating. Many people struggle with guilt or shame after eating certain foods, leading to a negative relationship with food and their bodies. Mindfulness teaches you to be compassionate with yourself, letting go of guilt and focusing on making balanced choices without harsh self-criticism. This mindset shift fosters a more sustainable, healthy approach to eating.

- **Practical Tip**: If you indulge in a less nutritious meal or snack, practice self-compassion. Remind yourself that one meal doesn't define your overall progress, and focus on making the next choice a healthier one.

Simple Mindfulness and Meditation Exercises to Curb Cravings and Manage Stress

Mindfulness and meditation offer practical techniques to help you manage cravings, reduce stress, and stay focused on your weight loss journey. Here are a few exercises that can be easily integrated into your daily routine:

1. Mindful Eating Exercise

One of the simplest and most effective mindfulness practices for weight loss is mindful eating. This exercise involves paying close attention to the sensory experience of eating—how the food looks, smells, tastes, and feels in your mouth. It helps slow down the eating process and increases your awareness of satiety signals, preventing overeating.

- **How to Practice**:
  - Before you begin eating, take a deep breath and set the intention to eat mindfully.
  - As you take each bite, focus on the taste, texture, and aroma of the food. Chew slowly, and notice the sensations in your body.
  - Pause between bites, putting down your fork, and check in with your hunger levels throughout the meal. Stop eating when you feel satisfied, not overly full.

2. Craving Meditation

When a craving strikes, it can feel overwhelming and difficult to resist. Instead of immediately giving in or using willpower to fight it, a craving meditation can help you observe the craving without acting on it. This mindfulness exercise allows you to sit with the discomfort of the craving and let it pass.

- **How to Practice**:
    - When you experience a craving, find a quiet place to sit and close your eyes. Take a few deep breaths.
    - Acknowledge the craving without judgment. Notice where you feel it in your body—maybe it's a tightness in your stomach or a sense of restlessness.
    - Instead of trying to suppress the craving, observe it. Allow the sensation to exist without giving in to it. Over time, you'll notice the craving diminishes.
    - Once the craving passes, take another deep breath and move on with your day without acting on it.

3. Body Scan Meditation for Stress Relief

Stress is one of the leading contributors to emotional eating and weight gain. The body scan meditation is a mindfulness practice that helps you become more aware of physical sensations, releasing tension and calming your mind. By reducing stress, you can prevent stress-induced overeating and make more mindful choices.

- **How to Practice**:
  - Find a quiet place to sit or lie down. Close your eyes and take a few deep breaths to center yourself.
  - Starting from the top of your head, bring your attention to each part of your body, slowly moving down to your feet. Notice any areas of tension or discomfort, and

> simply observe without trying to change anything.

- o As you continue, take deep breaths and imagine sending relaxation to each part of your body.
- o Finish the practice by taking a few deep, calming breaths, and bring your awareness back to the present moment.

The Role of Deep Breathing, Yoga, and Relaxation Techniques in Maintaining Focus

In addition to meditation, incorporating deep breathing, yoga, and relaxation techniques into your routine can further enhance mindfulness and support your weight loss goals. These practices not only calm the mind but also increase body awareness, helping you stay in tune with your body's needs.

1. Deep Breathing for Stress Management

Deep breathing exercises are simple yet powerful tools for reducing stress and anxiety, which are common triggers for overeating. By slowing down your breath, you activate your parasympathetic nervous system, which promotes relaxation and helps you make more mindful choices.

- **Practical Tip**: When you feel overwhelmed or stressed, practice deep breathing by inhaling slowly through your nose for a count of four, holding your breath for a count of four, and exhaling slowly through your mouth for a count of four. Repeat this process for several minutes to calm your mind and body.

2. Yoga for Mind-Body Awareness

Yoga is a physical practice that incorporates mindfulness, breath control, and movement, making it an excellent tool for weight loss. By increasing body awareness, yoga helps you tune into your physical and emotional states, making it easier to differentiate between emotional and physical hunger. It also reduces stress and promotes relaxation, which can prevent emotional eating.

- **Practical Tip**: Start with a simple yoga practice, focusing on poses that promote relaxation and mindfulness, such as child's pose, downward dog, and seated forward bends. As you move through the poses, focus on your breath and the sensations in your body, staying present in each movement.

3. *Progressive Muscle Relaxation*

Progressive muscle relaxation is a technique that involves tensing and then relaxing different muscle groups in the body. This practice helps release physical tension and reduce stress, making it a helpful tool for managing cravings and emotional triggers.

- **Practical Tip**: Find a quiet place to sit or lie down. Starting with your toes, tense the muscles in your feet for five seconds, then release the tension and focus on the sensation of relaxation. Gradually move up through your body, tensing and relaxing each muscle group until you reach your head. This practice can help calm your mind and reduce the urge to turn to food for comfort.

Real-Life Examples of People Using Mindfulness for Weight Loss Success

The power of mindfulness for weight loss is not just theoretical—it has helped countless individuals break free from unhealthy eating habits and develop a healthier relationship with food. Here are a few examples of people who have successfully used mindfulness techniques to achieve their weight loss goals:

1. Sarah's Story: Breaking Free from Emotional Eating

Sarah had struggled with emotional eating for years, often turning to food to cope with stress from her demanding job. She knew that her eating habits were sabotaging her weight loss efforts, but she felt powerless to stop. After learning about mindfulness, Sarah began practicing mindful eating and meditation daily. Over time, she became more aware of her emotional triggers and learned to respond to stress with deep breathing and relaxation techniques rather than food. Through mindfulness, Sarah was able to lose 20 pounds and maintain her weight loss by building a healthier relationship with food.

2. John's Story: Using Meditation to Overcome Cravings

John had always struggled with intense cravings for sugary snacks, which often derailed his weight loss efforts. After reading about the benefits of meditation for managing cravings, John started incorporating a craving meditation practice into his daily routine. Whenever he felt a craving, he would take a few minutes to meditate and observe the craving without acting on it. Over time, John found that his cravings became less frequent and intense, and he was able to stick to his healthy eating plan more consistently. John credits mindfulness and meditation with helping him lose 30 pounds and develop more discipline around food.

3. Emily's Story: Finding Balance with Yoga

Emily had tried various diets and exercise programs but struggled to maintain her weight loss because of her all-or-nothing mentality. After discovering yoga, Emily learned to approach weight loss with more balance and mindfulness. Through regular yoga practice, she became more attuned to her body's needs and found joy in movement for the first time. Yoga also helped Emily reduce stress and emotional eating, leading to a sustainable 15-pound weight loss. For Emily, yoga and mindfulness were key to transforming her relationship with her body and food.

Mindfulness as a Lifelong Tool for Weight Loss

Mindfulness and meditation are not quick fixes for weight loss—they are lifelong tools that can help you develop a healthier relationship with food, manage stress, and make more intentional choices about what you eat. By practicing mindfulness, you can break free from the cycle of emotional eating and cultivate a more balanced approach to weight loss that goes beyond the scale. Remember, weight loss is not just about what you eat but how you think and feel about food and your body. Mindfulness helps you bridge that gap, empowering you to make lasting, positive changes in your life.

As the saying goes, "The mind is everything. What you think, you become." By cultivating mindfulness and staying present in your weight loss journey, you can achieve your goals with greater clarity, focus, and self-compassion.

Chapter 12

Maintaining Long-Term Success: Life After Weight Loss

Losing weight is a significant achievement, but maintaining that weight loss over the long term can be an even greater challenge. Many people successfully shed pounds, only to struggle with keeping them off, facing the risk of regaining what they've worked so hard to lose. The reality is that maintaining weight loss requires a different mindset and set of strategies than those used to lose weight in the first place.

This chapter explores the psychology of maintaining weight loss, how to stay focused and avoid slipping back into old habits, and practical strategies for self-monitoring and accountability. We'll also look at how setting new health goals beyond weight loss can drive continued personal growth. Finally, we'll hear testimonials from individuals who have successfully maintained their weight loss over the years, offering real-life insights and inspiration.

The Psychology of Maintaining Weight Loss: Why It's Different from Losing Weight

The mindset required to maintain weight loss is different from the one that drives the weight loss process itself. When you're actively trying to lose weight, the goal is clear: reduce calories, increase activity, and see the numbers on the scale go down. There's a tangible reward each time you reach a milestone.

However, once you've achieved your weight loss goal, the immediate external motivator (seeing the scale drop) is gone, and the challenge becomes maintaining those healthy habits without the daily validation of weight loss progress. This transition requires shifting your focus from short-term goals to long-term lifestyle changes.

1. Sustaining Motivation Without a Visible Goal

One of the psychological hurdles in maintaining weight loss is that it's no longer about achieving something new but rather sustaining something already achieved. For many, this can feel less exciting and lead to a loss of motivation. Instead of aiming for a specific number on the scale, maintaining weight loss requires an internal motivation to live a healthy, balanced life.

- **Practical Tip**: Reframe your thinking from "I need to keep losing weight" to "I am committed to staying healthy and strong for life." Celebrate the progress you've made and shift your focus from the scale to how you feel—your energy levels, fitness, and overall well-being.

2. Understanding Set Point Theory

Set point theory suggests that your body has a natural weight range it tries to maintain, influenced by genetics, hormones, and metabolism. After significant weight loss, your body may resist maintaining a lower weight by increasing hunger hormones and slowing metabolism. Understanding this can help you approach weight maintenance with greater compassion for yourself and the need for ongoing vigilance.

- **Practical Tip**: Be aware of your body's signals, and stay proactive about managing your weight. Keep up with your exercise routines and mindful eating habits, but don't be discouraged by slight fluctuations. Focus on how your clothes fit and how you feel rather than obsessing over every pound on the scale.

How to Stay Focused and Avoid Falling Back into Old Habits

One of the biggest challenges after weight loss is avoiding the trap of slipping back into old habits. It's easy to feel complacent once you've reached your goal, but maintenance requires continued effort and attention. Fortunately, there are effective strategies to help you stay focused and avoid regaining weight.

1. Avoid the "Finish Line" Mentality

Many people approach weight loss with a mindset of "I'll do this until I reach my goal." However, thinking of weight loss as a temporary endeavor can lead to falling back into old patterns once the goal is reached. To maintain your success, it's essential to view healthy eating and regular exercise as permanent, lifelong habits.

- **Practical Tip**: Create a sustainable routine that includes enjoyable activities and foods you love, so maintaining your healthy lifestyle doesn't feel like a chore. Don't go back to old eating habits, even if you allow for occasional indulgences.

2. Establish a Routine That Supports Long-Term Success

The most successful weight maintainers are those who establish routines that fit their lifestyle and are enjoyable enough to stick with. Routines provide structure and prevent you from falling into impulsive or unhealthy behaviors.

- **Practical Tip**: Develop a consistent schedule for meals, exercise, and sleep. Having regular times for eating and activity can help you avoid overeating or skipping workouts. Plan your meals and workouts at the beginning of each week to create a sense of accountability.

3. Recognize Emotional and Stress Triggers

Just as in the weight loss phase, emotional eating, stress, and boredom can lead to overeating during maintenance. It's important to continue recognizing and managing these triggers, using the tools you developed during your weight loss journey.

- **Practical Tip**: Keep practicing mindfulness techniques, such as mindful eating and stress management exercises, to stay aware of your emotional states. When you feel the urge to eat for emotional reasons, pause and ask yourself if you're truly hungry or if there's another emotion at play. If it's stress or boredom, try to address those feelings in other ways, such as going for a walk or practicing deep breathing.

Strategies for Ongoing Self-Monitoring and Accountability

Maintaining weight loss requires continuous self-monitoring and accountability, both to yourself and to others. While it's natural to relax some of the strictness that comes with active weight loss, maintaining awareness of your habits is essential for long-term success.

1. Regular Self-Weighing and Monitoring

Research shows that individuals who weigh themselves regularly are more successful at maintaining their weight loss. Regular self-weighing keeps you aware of any potential weight gain and allows you to take corrective action before small gains turn into larger ones. However, it's important not to become overly fixated on the scale.

- **Practical Tip**: Weigh yourself once a week rather than daily. This provides a regular check-in without becoming obsessive. In addition to weighing yourself, keep an eye on how your clothes fit and how you feel overall.

2. Food Journaling

Even after losing weight, keeping track of what you eat can be a powerful tool for maintaining your success. A food journal helps you stay mindful of your food choices, portion sizes, and any emotional eating tendencies.

- **Practical Tip**: Continue to log your meals and snacks, either in a notebook or with an app. This doesn't mean you need to track every calorie, but it helps you stay conscious of your eating habits. You can also note your emotions and hunger levels alongside your meals to identify any patterns.

3. Accountability Partners and Support Networks

Accountability is crucial in maintaining weight loss. Whether it's a friend, family member, or online community, having people who support your healthy lifestyle can keep you on track. They can offer encouragement, share tips, and help you navigate challenges.

- **Practical Tip**: Partner with someone who shares your goals or join a weight maintenance group, either in person or online. Regularly check in with your accountability partner to discuss your progress, celebrate successes, and talk through any challenges.

How to Set New, Non-Weight-Related Health Goals for Continued Personal Growth

One of the keys to long-term weight maintenance is shifting your focus from the scale to other areas of health and personal growth. Setting new goals that aren't solely focused on weight can help you stay motivated and engaged in your health journey.

1. Focus on Fitness and Strength Goals

Now that you've reached your weight loss goal, consider focusing on fitness goals like improving your strength, endurance, or flexibility. Setting goals related to physical performance can keep you excited about your workouts and give you a new sense of accomplishment.

- **Practical Tip**: Set specific fitness goals, such as running a certain distance, lifting a specific amount of weight, or mastering a yoga pose. Celebrate these achievements just as you would celebrate weight loss milestones.

2. Prioritize Mental and Emotional Health

Maintaining your mental and emotional well-being is just as important as maintaining your physical health. Set goals related to stress management, mindfulness, and overall happiness. These can help you stay balanced and prevent emotional eating or unhealthy habits from creeping back in.

- **Practical Tip**: Incorporate practices like meditation, journaling, or therapy into your routine to support your mental health. Setting goals related to reducing stress or increasing your mindfulness can enhance your overall quality of life.

3. Set Nutritional Goals Beyond Weight Loss

Once the focus is no longer on calorie restriction, you can shift your attention to nourishing your body with the healthiest foods possible. Consider setting goals related to trying new recipes, increasing your intake of fruits and vegetables, or experimenting with new cooking techniques.

- **Practical Tip**: Set weekly or monthly goals, such as trying one new healthy recipe each week or incorporating more plant-based meals into your diet. These goals keep you engaged with your food choices without the pressure of weight loss.

Testimonials: Stories of Long-Term Weight Loss Maintenance

Hearing from others who have successfully maintained their weight loss can provide inspiration and practical insights. Here are a few stories of individuals who have not only achieved weight loss but have also maintained it over the long term.

1. Emma's Story: Finding Balance After Weight Loss

Emma lost 50 pounds over the course of a year but found maintaining that loss was a new challenge. She realized that she needed to shift her focus from strict dieting to a more balanced approach. Emma started setting fitness goals, such as running her first 5K, and began practicing mindfulness to stay present in her eating habits. Five years later, Emma has kept the weight off and continues to set new health goals to stay motivated.

2. Michael's Story: Accountability and Community Support

After losing 40 pounds, Michael knew he needed to stay accountable to keep the weight off. He joined a local fitness group where he made new friends who shared his goals. This community support kept him motivated, and he continued attending group workouts and social events that revolved around healthy living. Michael has maintained his weight loss for over three years and credits his accountability partners for helping him stay on track.

3. Sophia's Story: Setting New Goals for Growth

Sophia lost 30 pounds and initially struggled with weight maintenance, feeling like she had lost her purpose. She decided to set new goals unrelated to weight, such as improving her flexibility through yoga and learning more about nutrition. Sophia now focuses on how she feels rather than what the scale says, and she has maintained her weight loss for two years while feeling healthier and more empowered than ever.

Embracing a Healthy Lifestyle for Life

Maintaining weight loss is not just about avoiding weight regain—it's about embracing a healthy, balanced lifestyle that supports your long-term well-being. By shifting your focus from the scale to other areas of growth, practicing ongoing self-monitoring, and staying connected to a support network, you can continue to thrive long after reaching your weight loss goal.

Remember, weight loss maintenance is a lifelong journey, not a destination. The habits you've built, the resilience you've developed, and the community you've created will continue to support you on this path. As you move forward, keep setting new goals, celebrating your successes, and learning from your challenges. In doing so, you'll continue to grow not just in health, but in all areas of life.

As the saying goes, "Success is the sum of small efforts repeated day in and day out." By continuing to make small, intentional efforts every day, you can maintain your success and enjoy a healthier, more fulfilling life.

Chapter 15

Resources and Tools for Continued Success

Achieving and maintaining weight loss is not just about knowledge and motivation—it's also about having the right resources and tools to support your journey. In this chapter, we will provide you with a variety of recommendations, including books, podcasts, online communities, tracking tools, and practical worksheets to help you stay on course. These resources will not only help you monitor your progress but also offer ongoing inspiration and guidance as you continue working toward your health goals.

Recommended Books, Podcasts, and Online Resources

Knowledge is power, and the more you educate yourself about weight loss, nutrition, and mindset, the better equipped you will be to navigate challenges and stay motivated. Below are some highly recommended resources that can further expand your understanding of the mental, physical, and emotional aspects of weight loss.

Books

1. **"Atomic Habits" by James Clear**
   This book is a must-read for anyone looking to create lasting change. It focuses on the science of habit formation and provides practical strategies for building good habits and breaking bad ones. Clear emphasizes the importance of small, consistent changes that lead to significant results over time—key principles for sustainable weight loss.

2. **"The Power of Now" by Eckhart Tolle**

   Tolle's book focuses on mindfulness and staying present, which can help you become more aware of your thoughts, feelings, and actions related to food and exercise. Practicing mindfulness can help you break the cycle of emotional eating and foster a healthier relationship with food.

3. **"The Obesity Code" by Dr. Jason Fung**

   This book dives into the science behind weight gain, insulin resistance, and metabolic health. Dr. Fung explains how intermittent fasting and proper nutrition can play key roles in weight loss, while also addressing the psychological aspects of overeating and dieting.

4. **"Mindful Eating" by Jan Chozen Bays**

Mindful eating is a powerful tool for weight management, and this book provides detailed guidance on how to become more aware of your eating habits. It teaches you to listen to your body's hunger cues and encourages a compassionate approach to eating without guilt or restriction.

Podcasts

1. **"The Model Health Show" with Shawn Stevenson**
Shawn Stevenson's podcast covers a wide range of health-related topics, from nutrition and exercise to mindset and personal growth. It's an excellent resource for anyone interested in improving their overall well-being through science-backed strategies.

2. **"The Mindset Mentor" with Rob Dial**
Weight loss is just as much about mental

discipline as it is about physical changes. Rob Dial's podcast is perfect for those looking to cultivate a stronger mindset, overcome limiting beliefs, and push through challenges. Episodes often focus on motivation, habit-building, and goal-setting—all critical components for weight loss success.

3. **"Food Psych" with Christy Harrison**
Focused on intuitive eating and dismantling diet culture, this podcast helps listeners develop a healthier relationship with food. Christy Harrison discusses topics such as body positivity, the psychology of eating, and how to free yourself from the endless cycle of dieting and emotional eating.

4. **"The Habit Coach" with Ashdin Doctor**
This podcast offers short, actionable episodes on building habits that support

various aspects of life, including weight loss, fitness, and overall health. Ashdin Doctor provides practical tips on how to develop consistency and discipline, helping you form sustainable habits that last.

Online Resources

1. **MyFitnessPal**

   A popular app for tracking calories, macronutrients, and physical activity, MyFitnessPal also includes a large community of users for added support. Its extensive food database makes it easy to log meals and monitor progress, while its social features allow you to connect with others on similar weight loss journeys.

2. **Lose It!**

   This is another excellent app for tracking your food intake, weight loss, and fitness goals. Lose It! also features meal planning tools, personalized goals, and the ability to scan barcodes for easy logging. It's a user-friendly platform that helps you stay accountable and organized.

3. **Healthline's Nutrition and Fitness Section**

   Healthline is a trusted source of science-backed health information. Their Nutrition and Fitness sections provide up-to-date articles on weight loss strategies, diet trends, exercise tips, and mental health. It's a great resource to continue learning about the latest research and advice on healthy living.

4. **Weight Loss Subreddit (r/loseit)**

   This Reddit community is a supportive space where people share their weight loss experiences, challenges, and victories. You can find motivation, ask questions, and connect with others who are on a similar journey. The community also offers a wealth of advice on everything from meal planning to emotional eating.

Weight Loss Tracking Tools: Apps and Journals to Monitor Progress

Tracking your progress is a key component of weight loss success. Whether you prefer digital tools or physical journals, staying accountable and monitoring your habits, food intake, and exercise routines can help you stay on track. Below are some of the best tools for tracking your weight loss journey.

1. MyFitnessPal

As mentioned earlier, MyFitnessPal is a comprehensive app for logging food, exercise, and weight. It offers daily reports and long-term insights into your eating patterns and nutritional intake. The app also allows you to set goals based on your individual needs, such as calorie intake, macronutrient ratios, or specific health objectives.

2. Fitbit

Fitbit not only tracks your physical activity but also integrates with food tracking apps like MyFitnessPal to provide a holistic view of your health. It monitors steps, sleep, heart rate, and exercise, making it an all-in-one solution for maintaining a healthy lifestyle.

3. HabitBull

If you're looking to track habits rather than calories, HabitBull is an excellent option. You can log habits related to food, exercise, hydration, sleep, and more. This app provides visual progress charts, reminders, and motivational quotes to help you stay consistent with your new healthy behaviors.

4. Pen and Paper Journal

For those who prefer a more tactile approach, a physical journal can be just as effective. Writing down your daily food intake, emotions, exercise routine, and reflections can help you stay mindful of your actions and choices. Journaling also allows for more personal reflection, helping you track your emotional and mental journey alongside the physical one.

5. The "Streaks" App

Streaks is a habit-tracking app that allows you to set and track up to 12 goals at a time. It's designed to help you build healthy habits by encouraging you to maintain "streaks" of consecutive days. This can be especially motivating when building new routines, like exercising daily or eating mindfully.

Helpful Worksheets and Exercises from the Book

Throughout this book, we've provided exercises to help you reflect on your progress, identify challenges, and set goals. Below are a few practical worksheets you can return to anytime you need to refocus or track your progress.

1. Limiting Beliefs Worksheet

In Chapter 2, we discussed how limiting beliefs can sabotage your weight loss efforts. Revisit the worksheet where you identified these beliefs, and update it with new insights or challenges you've faced since. Use the space to reframe any negative thoughts that arise as you progress through your journey.

2. Visualization and Goal-Setting Worksheet

From Chapter 6, this worksheet is designed to help you clarify your goals and visualize your success. Revisit your long-term goals regularly, and don't hesitate to adjust them based on your progress. Visualizing your success can keep you focused and motivated when challenges arise.

3. Mindful Eating Journal

Mindful eating is an important practice in weight management, and keeping a journal can help you track your eating habits, emotional triggers, and hunger cues. Reflect on how you feel before, during, and after meals to identify patterns that may be contributing to overeating or unhealthy food choices.

4. Exercise Routine Planner

Use this worksheet from Chapter 10 to create a structured, balanced exercise routine that works for your lifestyle. Break your goals into manageable weekly actions and adjust your routine as your fitness level improves. Remember to include activities that you enjoy, as this will help you stay consistent.

5. Accountability Partner Plan

Chapter 8 discussed the importance of building a support system. Use this worksheet to list potential accountability partners, online communities, or professional resources that can help you stay on track. Outline how and when you'll check in with them to maintain accountability and support.

Final Thoughts

Your journey to sustainable weight loss is deeply personal, but you don't have to go through it alone. With the right tools and resources, you can stay focused, motivated, and empowered to achieve lasting change. Whether you turn to apps, books, podcasts, or support networks, remember that progress is ongoing—and it's okay to seek help when you need it.

Ultimately, the tools you choose should align with your lifestyle, values, and preferences. Find what works best for you, and use these resources to stay engaged, accountable, and inspired as you continue on your journey to a healthier, happier life. Keep learning, keep growing, and remember: small steps lead to significant, lasting change. You have everything you need to succeed—one step at a time.